A. Gullo • P.D. Lumb (Eds.)

Intensive and Critical Care Medicine
Reflections, Recommendations and Perspectives

W0227938

A. Gullo • P.D. Lumb (Eds.)

Intensive and Critical Care Medicine

Reflections, Recommendations and Perspectives

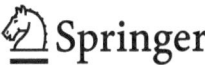 Springer

ANTONINO GULLO
Department of Perioperative Medicine
Intensive Care and Emergency
Trieste University School of Medicine
Trieste, Italy

PHILIP D. LUMB
Department of Anaesthesiology
Keck School of Medicine at USC
Los Angeles, CA
U.S.A.

Library of Congress Control Number: 2005928163

ISBN 88-470-0349-0 Springer Milan Berlin Heidelberg New York

Springer is a part of Springer Science+Business Media

springeronline.com

© Springer-Verlag Italia 2005

Printed in Italy

Cover design: Simona Colombo, Milan, Italy
Typesetting: Graphostudio, Milan, Italy
Printing: Arti Grafiche Stella, Trieste, Italy

Ten Steps to the Top

After the Sydney meeting held in 2001, the World Federation of Societies of Intensive and Critical Care Medicine (WFSICCM) reinforced its multidisciplinary and multi-professional identity.

WFSICCM President Philip D. Lumb from the Keck School of Medicine of the University of Southern California in Los Angeles has, together with the Federation Council, envisaged a new strategy to obtain a more-visible target for its mission.

In the last four years, several goals have been accomplished and the WFSICCM is now well-positioned to succeed in its global mission.

– First, the functions of the Secretariat and Headquarters have been relocated to the United Kingdom. Ms Liz Taylor has been appointed the Council's Executive Assistant, which represents a significant step towards ensuring the organisation's administrative integrity. Clearly, this is a winning decision;

– Second, the WF web-site has improved global communications and become a useful tool for effective online decision-making;

– Third, Pathfinder UK has helped to develop a strong marketing plan and to create a more-visible and proactive presence in the international Critical Care community;

– Fourth, the President has reached all corners of the world, communicating enthusiasm and revealing leadership excellence;

– Fifth, the Pan American and Iberian Federation of Societies of Intensive and Critical Care Medicine has reinforced its relationship with the World Federation; the memorable 2003 congress held in Cancun, Mexico, has represented a keystone in the growing process of the WF;

– Sixth, Trieste, Italy, has for three times hosted the WF during APICE, the International Congress endorsed by the WF;

– Seventh, Durban, South Africa, has represented an important phase in the expansion process of the WF; an important debate for understanding possible assistance for countries with limited resources has taken place there;

– Eighth, the Council has encouraged new contacts; the dream of establishing the Mediterranean School of Intensive and Critical Care Medicine is coming true.

Furthermore, Russia and China represent a new target for the WF Council, with scientific contacts and expectations becoming increasingly promising;

– Ninth, last April, in Santos, the WF Council considered the future scenario of the WF after the forthcoming 9th World Congress to be held in Buenos Aires; in the meantime, the capital of tango and the South American atmosphere will be an ideal environment for continuing our dreams;

– Tenth, Education and Standards of Care are the pillars of the WFSICCM; the present book is a celebration of the WF Council's quadrennial activity and sets out the reflections and perspectives that are necessary for offering care to the highest standards to critically ill patients. We hope we all agree to think about this.

Buenos Aires   *Antonino Gullo*
August 27, 2005   *Philip D. Lumb*

Table of Contents

List of Contributors

Azoulay E.
Intensive Care Unit,
Hôpital Saint Louis,
Paris (France)

Berggren L.
Department of Anaesthesiology,
Örebro Medical Centre Hospital,
Örebro (Sweden)

Besso J.
Department of Intensive Care,
Hospital Centro Medico de Caracas
(Venezuela)

Bhagwanjee S.
Department of Anaesthesiology,
University of Withwatersrand,
Johannesburg Hospital, Johannesburg
(South Africa)

de Latorre F.J.
Servei de Medicina Intensiva, Hospital
Universitari Vall d'Hebron, Barcelona
(Spain)

Dobb G.J.
Intensive Care Unit, Royal Perth
Hospital and School of Medicine and
Pharmacology, University of Western
Australia, Perth (Australia)

Dominguez-Cherit G.
Department of Critical Care Medicine,
National Institute of Medical Sciences
and Nutrition 'Salvador Zubiran',
Mexico City (Mexico)

Fisher M.
Intensive Care Unit, Royal North Shore
Hospital, St. Leonards (Australia)

Gallesio A.O.
Unidad de Terapia Intensiva Adulta,
Hospital Italiano, Buenos Aires
(Argentina)

Gullo A.
Department of Perioperative
Medicine, Intensive Care and
Emergency, School of Anaesthesia and
Intensive Care, Trieste University
Medical School, Trieste (Italy)

Gutierrez J.
Department of Critical Care Medicine,
National Institute of Medical Sciences
and Nutrition 'Salvador Zubiran',
Mexico City (Mexico)

Iscra F.
Department of Perioperative
Medicine, Intensive Care and
Emergency, School of Anaesthesia and

Intensive Care, Trieste University
Medical School, Trieste (Italy)

Jahagirdar A.
Shree Medical Foundation, Prayag
Hospital, Pune (India)

Le Gall J.R.
Intensive Care Unit, Hôpital Saint
Louis, Paris (France)

Lumb P.D.
Department of Anaesthesiology, Keck
School of Medicine, University of
Southern California, Los Angeles
(USA)

Mello Moreira M.
Department of Surgery, Faculdade de
Ciências Médicas, Universidade
Estadual de Campinas UNICAMP,
Campinas, São Paulo (Brazil)

Metnitz P.
Department of Anaesthesiology and
Intensive Care Medicine, Medical
University of Vienna, Vienna (Austria)

Moreno R.
Unidade de Cuidados Intensivos
Polivalente, Hospital de Santo António
dos Capuchos, Centro Hospitalar de
Lisboa, Lisbon (Portugal)

Padron J.
Department of Intensive Care, Hospital
Centro Medico de Caracas (Venezuela)

Plaz J.
Department of Intensive Care, Hospital
Centro Medico de Caracas (Venezuela)

Prayag S.
Shree Medical Foundation, Prayag
Hospital, Pune (India)

Pru C.
Department of Intensive Care, Hospital
Centro Medico de Caracas (Venezuela)

Rivero E.
Department of Critical Care Medicine,
National Institute of Medical Sciences
and Nutrition 'Salvador Zubiran',
Mexico City (Mexico)

Rubulotta F.
Department of Intensive Care,
University Hospital, Leuven (Belgium)

Takezawa J.
Department of Emergency and
Intensive Care Medicine, Nagoya
University School of Medicine, Nagoya
(Japan)

Terzi R.
Department of Surgery, Faculdade de
Ciências Médicas, Universidade
Estadual de Campinas UNICAMP,
Campinas, São Paulo (Brazil)

Williams G.
Direction of Nursing, Maroondah
Hospital, Victoria (Australia)

Williams T.A.
Intensive Care Unit, Royal Perth
Hospital and School of Medicine and
Pharmacology, University of Western
Australia, Perth (Australia)

Abbreviations

A	Adenine
ACTH	Adrenocorticotropic Hormone
ADE	Adverse Drug Effects
AIDS	Acquired Immunodeficiency Syndrome
APACHE	Acute Physiology and Chronic Health Evaluation
APC	Antigen Presenting Cell
APS	Acute Physiology Score
ARDS	Acute Respiratory Distress Syndrome
ARF	Acute Respiratory Failure
ARV	Anti-retroviral
BIPAP	Biphasic Positive Air Pressure
C	Cytosine
CAM	Cell Adhesion Molecules
CAP	Community Acquired Pneumonia
CARS	Compensatory Anti-Inflammatory Response Syndrome
CDC	Centers for Disease Control and Prevention
CI	Confidence Interval
CMV	Cytomegalovirus
COPD	Chronic Obstructive Pulmonary Disease
CPAP	Continuous Positive Airway Pressure
CPI	Consumer Price Index
CPR	Cardiopulmonary Resuscitation
CR-BIS	Catheter-Related Blood Stream Infection
CVVH	Continuous Veno-Venous Haemofiltration
DD	D-Dimer
DHEA	Dheydroepiandrosterone
DIC	Disseminated Intravascular Coagulation
DISC	Death-Inducing Signalling Complex
DNA	Deoxyribonucleic Acid
DNAR	Do Not Attempt Resuscitation
DNR	Do Not Resuscitate

DVT	Deep Venous Thrombosis
EGDT	Early Goal Directed Therapy
ENAS	European-North American Study
EPIC	European Prospective Infection Control
ER	Emergency Room
FGF	Fibroplastic Growth Factor
FRC	Functional Residual Capacity
FVC	Forced Vital Capacity
G	Guanine
GFR	Glomerular Filtration Rate
HIPPA	Healthcare Information Portability and Privacy Act
HR	Hazard Ratio
HR	Heart Rate
HRS	Hepatorenal Syndrome
I/R	Ischaemic Reperfusion Injury
ICD	International Classification of Diseases
ICP	Intracranial Pressure
ICU	Intensive Care Unit
IPAP	Inspiratory Positive Air Pressure
IRB	Institutional Revue Board
JANIS	Japanese Nosocomial Infection Surveillance
JCAHO	Joint Commission on Accreditation of Heathcare Organizations
LPS	Lipoproteins
MARS	Molecular Adsorbent Recirculating System
MI	Myocardial Infarction
MODS	Multiple Organ Dysfunction Syndrome
MPM	Mortality Probability Models
MPTP	Mitochondrial Permeability Transition
mRNA	Messenger Ribonucleic Acid
NAC	N-acetylcysteine
NAS	Nursing Activity Score
NIV	Non-Invasive Ventilation
NK	Natural Killer
NNIS	Nosocomial Infection Surveillance
NO	Nitrous oxide
NPPV	Non-invasive Positive Pressure Ventilation
NSAID	Nonsteroidal Anti-Inflammatory Drug
PaCO2	Partial Arterial Carbon Dioxide Pressure
PAD	Public Access Defibrillation
PAV	Proportional Assist Ventilation

PCP	Pneumocystis Carinii Pneumonia
PE	Pulmonary Embolism
PEEP	Positive End Expiratory Pressure
PIOPED	Prospective Investigators of Pulmonary Embolism Diagnosis
PRR	Pattern Recognition Receptor
QALY	Quality-Adjusted Life-Year
RAAS	Renin-Angiotensin-Aldosterone System
RNA	Ribonucleic Acid
ROC	Receiver Operating Characteristic
ROS	Reactive Oxygen Species
RPF	Renal Plasma Flow
rRNA	Ribosomal Ribonucleic Acid
SAPS	Simplified Acute Physiology Score
SBP	Spontaneous Bacterial Peritonitis
SCCM	Society of Critical Care Medicine
SDD	Selective Digestive Decontamination
SIRS	Systemic Inflammatory Response Syndrome
SMR	Standard Mortality Ration
SNP	Single Nucleotide Polymorphism
SNS	Sympathetic Nervous System
SOD	Superoxide Dismutase
SOFA	Sepsis-Related Organ Failure Assessment
SP	Standard of Practice
SSI	Surgical Site Infection
SUPPORT	Study to Understand Prognoses and Preferences for Outcomes and Risk of Treatment
SvO2	Oxygen Venous Saturation
T	Thymine
TB	Tuberculosis
TEE	Trans-oesophageal Echocardiography
TIPS	Transjugular Intrahepatic Stent-Shunt
TISS	Therapeutic Intervention Scoring System
TLR4	Toll-Like Receptor 4
tRNA	Transfer Ribonucleic Acid
UTI	Urinary Catheter-related Infection
V/Q	Ventilation Perfusion Ratio
VAP	Ventialtor Associated Pneumonia
V_D/V_T phys	Physiologic Dead Space
VNTR	Variable Number of Tandem Repeats
WFSICCM	World Federation of Societies of Intensive and Critical Care Medicine

Council of the WFSICCM

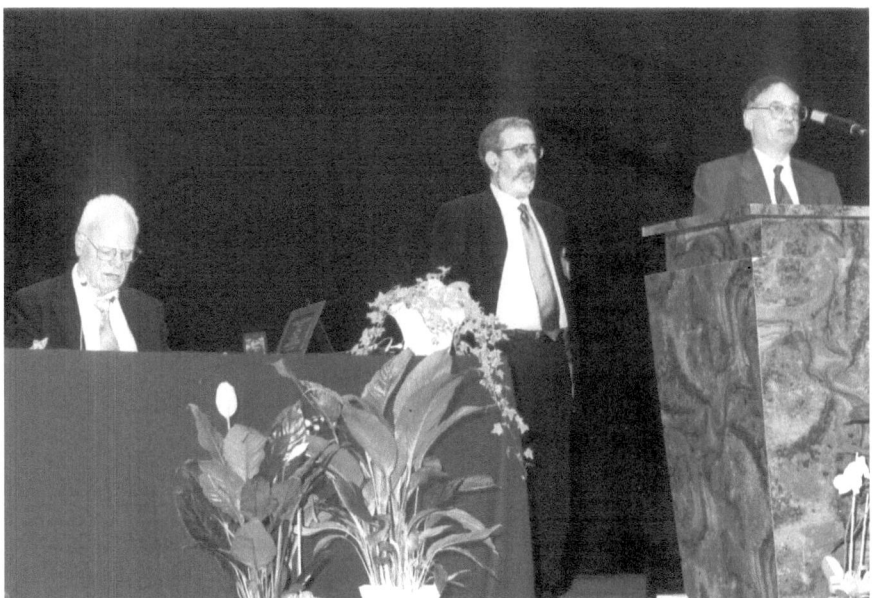

Left to right: A. Gilston (UK) *First President WFSICCM*, A. Gullo (Italy), W.C. Shoemaker (USA); Trieste, Welcome Ceremony, APICE 1998

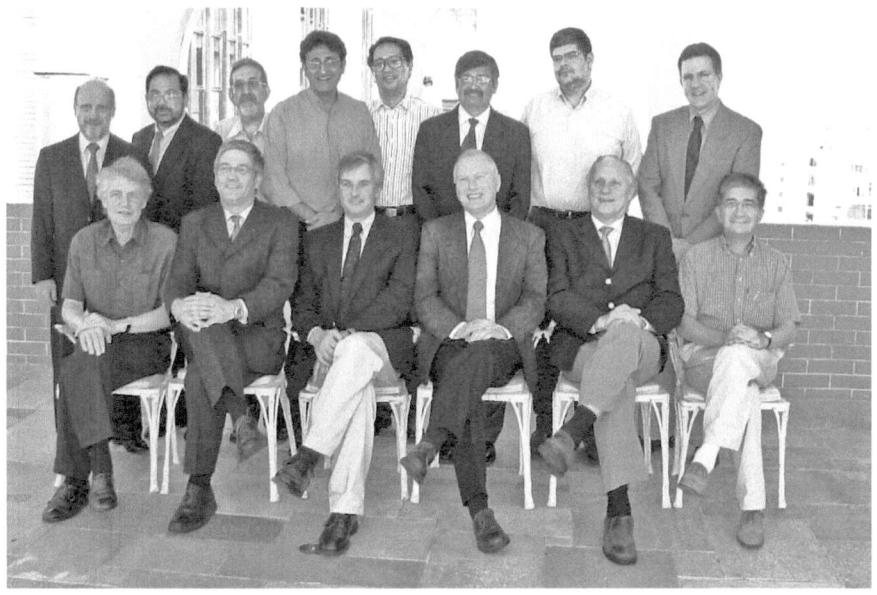

WFSICCM Board in Santos, April 2005 - Left to right, stand: A. Gallesio (Argentina), J. Besso (Venezuela), A. Gullo (Italy), S. Bhagwanjee (South Africa), J. Takezawa (Japan), S. Prayag (India), R.P.J. Moreno (Portugal), G. Williams (Australia)
Sit: L. Berggren (Sweden), G. Park (UK), P.D. Lumb (USA), G.J. Dobb (Australia), R.G.G. Terzi (Brazil), J.R. Le Gall (France)

Introduction: World Federation 1993-1997

M. FISHER

At the 1993 World Congress of the Federation in Madrid I was elected President of the World Federation. The Secretary General was Christopher Bryan Brown of the United States and the Treasurer was Dr David Ryan of the United Kingdom. It immediately became apparent that we had no Executive Member from the new elected delegates, which would cause a problem when the Executive changed 4 years later.

The 4-year period for which I was President was characterised as a period of little growth in the Federation as we endeavoured with some difficulty in keeping the organisation afloat.

The publishing company King and Wirth had a long and successful association with the society which gave them access to the society's mailing list and in return lead to a financial payment to the Federation and the production of the journal 'Intensive Care World'. This journal was the Federation's flagship and the only intensive care literature received by many of the member societies throughout the world. King and Wirth were no longer willing and able to continue to provide these services. The directors of King and Wirth set out to find an alternative group to take over the publishing and the mailing list activities of the Federation. They arranged a number of preliminary discussions between myself and members of suitable companies which eventually led to council approving an agreement signed with Mr David Campbell at the World Congress in Ottawa. Mr Campbell ran a successful medical publishing company called Global HealthCare Communications. This relationship promised many exciting opportunities for the Federation, particularly with respect to broadband communication. Over the time I was associated with the Federation, the increasing use of the Internet and e-mail for transmission of information had made a major improvement in the ability to communicate within council. Global HealthCare Communications was interested in taking electronic communication further with real-time broadcasting of intensive care symposia to members and in electronic publication of the journal, and creation of a website. Luciano Gattinoni was able to obtain a generous grant from Mallinckrodt to establish a website. Unfortunately, our relationship with Global was not a happy one: the journal did not survive and the website was unsatisfactory. Global was sold to another company and to all intents and purposes disappeared. The problems will no doubt be dealt with in subsequent chapters.

The second problem the Executive had to confront was that Ms Rika Sevy, who had been the Secretary and Business Manager, and a tireless champion of the Federation since its inception had to resign for personal reasons. We sought tenders from member societies to administer the business of the Federation. It was agreed at a council meeting in 1995 that the offer from the Intensive Care Society (UK) should be accepted. This then became a permanent home of the World Federation.

The only other problems encountered during the period 1993-1997 were those over membership. This generally revolved around conflicts between the two societies as to who would be the official representative of the country. In the case of the two Indian societies it was agreed that both could be members. This was strenuously resisted by the President of the original society, Dr N.P. Singh, who was a very active member of the Federation. However, Dr Singh's society vanished over subsequent years and the Indian Society for Critical Care Medicine became an active member.

A request for membership from a Greek society encompassing both anaesthesia and intensive care was opposed by the Hellenic Society which was solely an intensive care society. The Hellenic Society was invited to apply for membership at the Toronto World Congress but demanded that the Macedonian Society be expelled prior to the Hellenic Society's entry. This was neither possible within the constitution nor appropriate in the opinion of council.

Other political problems occurred in relationship to the Sydney World Congress and it is important in my opinion that a World Federation does all it can to ensure it is a body for doctors (and nurses) and not involved in problems which are not able to be influenced by the organisation, nor relevant to the majority of members.

Throughout the course of my presidency, the Federation's financial position was precarious in spite of the excellent and diligent stewardship of treasurer David Ryan. Revenue from the Madrid meeting was lower than expected and the loss of King and transition to the new headquarters reduced the ability to collect subscriptions. We minimised costs by meeting in association with other congresses and providing speakers in return for a meeting venue and accommodation. Our thanks for support in these activities go to the Pan-Iberian Society, SCCM , and Jean Louis Vincent.

Efforts to improve the society's financial position, particularly in the light of losing the income from publishing and membership activities were largely unsuccessful.

Prior to the Intensive Care Meeting in Ottawa, we were able to attract Ms Sevy back to the society and were able to facilitate the transfer of the society's records and archives to the Intensive Care Society (UK). Ms Sevy was available to run the Federation's business at the Toronto Congress, which was a great relief to the council. Dr Luciano Gattinoni became the new president of the Federation in Toronto.

Because of a lack of corporate knowledge in the new Executive, I was asked to remain n as an ex-officio member and was associated with the executive activities up until the World Congress of 2001.

One of the philosophies we tried to support in Council was helping people from developing countries. The World Federation sponsored a number of delegates by paying their registration to attend the World Congress held in Ottawa in 1997. However, the World Federation's arrangement with the Canadian Society meant that the entire share of the profits made by the World Federation was to be taken up by the sponsored registrations. The Canadian Society of Critical Care very graciously took over the cost of the registrations themselves.

The World Congress in 2001 marked a major landmark in the society's activities. While a number of other World Congress meetings had made small profits and the Canadian meeting made a reasonable profit, the Australian meeting made a substantial profit despite spending a great deal more on social functions and other activities than previously. The Australian and New Zealand Intensive Care Society was able to increase the World Federation's share of the profit by 50% more than the agreement. Major efforts were made with the 2001 meeting to change some of the previous ways of doing things. All the invited speakers were required to pay fees to the Federation for the cost of accommodation and registration. Accommodation and living allowances were provided to a number of people who would otherwise have been unable to come and we were able to sponsor people from South America, Cuba, Vietnam and Nepal. A number of nurses from Malawi and Rwanda were also able to attend and remain in Sydney to gain experience in intensive care units, and in association with various other groups, a number of other people were able to remain in Australia and New Zealand for training. There were a number of sponsored people who were unable to attend because of the difficulty in getting visas after the World Trade Centre attacks on the 11th September 2001. Indeed although this led to a number of cancellations of speaking delegates at the meeting, particularly from Portugal and the United States, the over 2000 registrations meant that the meeting did not suffer in a major way from these cancellations. The opening ceremony has passed into legend: it seemed to us that most opening ceremonies are the same and the speeches the same too. Our only speakers were patients and relatives and with one exception (a patient), the solo artists were all doctors and nurses. The ceremony was held together by the Sydney Gay and Lesbian Choir.

We were conscious when running this meeting of a complete lack of corporate history in terms of what had gone on before and at the end of the meeting a CD was produced containing advice and details of budgets and tender documents, etc., for future organisers of the meeting.

Overall, my term as President was associated with little growth and problem-solving and we were unable to hand over a Federation that fulfilled our goals to the new executive.

Consent and Intensive Care: Is It Possible?

L. Berggren

The intensive care environment is complex and sometimes confusing to both patients and their relatives. Decisions concerning diagnosis, treatment, and prognosis are often made in emergency situations with insufficient underlying information. Also, the clinical situation sometimes imposes great strain upon the intensive care physician and the assisting team. The discussion of different potential treatment options with relatives or patients might thus be both difficult and stressful and not the main priority. Furthermore, most patients admitted to the intensive care unit (ICU) are not competent and a priori excluded from any possibility of autonomous decision making. Today, in medical practice in general, there is a shift from paternalism towards shared decision making. Also, legislation in many countries mandates informed consent. The problems in the ICU setting are obvious. When and what to tell patients and relatives can be contentious issues and are influenced by the physician's beliefs, knowledge, and attitudes just as much as more objective patient factors, making the situation even harder in clinical ICU practice.

Meaning of Informed Consent

Informed consent is the process by which a person authorises medical treatment after discussion with clinicians regarding the nature, indications, benefits, and risks of treatment [1]. It has obvious ethical and legal implications. There are three broad aspects of intensive care practice for which consent is relevant. The first relates to invasive procedures, the second to treatment and diagnosis options and strategies, and the third to research participation. The third aspect, however important, is beyond the scope of this paper. As previously stated, consent is often and regularly given by relatives or proxies. More than half of all consents were given by proxies in a recent study from a North

American university ICU. This did not change after an intervention with introduction of a standardised consent form [2]. However, it is an open question as to what extent surrogate decision making actually reflects the will of the patient, especially in an emotionally stressful situation. The problem might not be that difficult when physicians are considering consent to common routine procedures, but it's immense when they are dealing with end-of-life issues. Another problem with surrogate decision making is the identification of the surrogates. Who are actually the surrogates? There are obvious personal, cultural, and societal differences concerning the preferences and recognition of proxies. Thus, surrogate decision making in the ICU is ultimately also a question of moral and ethical justification.

There are certain problems with obtaining consent for routine procedures. How to act if the surrogates refuse to allow the placing of a necessary central line for the safe delivery of vasoactive drugs? Are the relatives also able to refuse an arterial line or the appropriate antibiotic regimen? Clearly this approach has the potential to collapse into absurdity [3].

Consent for Commonly Performed Procedures

Consent to routine or everyday invasive procedures is often presumed under the general consent to ICU treatment. This is clearly not always the case. The practice differs substantially between and within countries. A recent study from the United States showed no uniform practice of consent for commonly performed invasive procedures between 173 ICU training program directors. The rate of consent for vascular access procedures ranged from 20 to 90%. The rates of obtaining consent for Foley catheterisation or nasogastric intubation was less than 10%. Consent was routinely obtained for GI endoscopy, bronchoscopy, and medical research [4]. The situation in Europe is the same, with a wide variation in practice between countries. In a postal survey, Vincent showed that 50% of ICU physicians required written informed consent for surgery, but only a few required consent for routine procedures like arterial lines. There were significant differences between different countries. The ICU physicians from Northern Europe, the Netherlands, and Scandinavia were more likely to accept 'no' or only oral consent for procedures, while German and British ones preferred written consent. Another interesting finding was that only 32% of ICU physicians would provide full information on an iatrogenic incident, but more than 70% felt they actually should. Again, geographically there were significant differences between doctors from the Netherlands and Scandinavia who were more likely to give complete information, and those from Greece, Spain, and Italy who were less likely [5]. The conclusion was that ICU physicians were not completely honest with their

patients regarding diagnosis, prognosis, or in the event of an iatrogenic incident. The practice of informed consent also varies substantially within
Europe. The situation outside these western countries is not clear. Data from
other regions of the world were lacking.

Willingness to Participate in Critical Decision Making

The principle of autonomy implies not only knowledge of problems and alternatives in the ICU setting, but also a pronounced willingness to take an active
part in decisions not only concerning routine procedures but also in real and
difficult end-of-life situations. This participation can not automatically be
taken for granted. The paternalistic approach, commonly viewed as oldfash-
ioned, holds the doctor as the sole decision maker and lifts the burden of
problematic decisions from the patients and their proxies. A situation actually appreciated by a few patients, particularly older and uninformed persons.
However, the principle of autonomy has gained increasing importance. In
most medical systems, it is the leading ethical principle. It implies the respect
for the deliberate choices made by persons in accordance with their own values. However, the paternalistic approach is still favoured by many doctors.
There are certain discrepancies between the attitudes of the general public,
ICU nurses, and ICU physicians towards end-of-life decisions as expressed in
a Swedish nation-wide postal survey. The majority of ICU physicians viewed
themselves as the sole decision makers. A view not supported by the nurses or
the public. The nurses and the public advocated a joint decision [6]. Even in
less dramatic decisions, the paternalistic approach is still favoured by many
doctors. The conclusion is that ICU physicians must increasingly be prepared
to involve both nurses and relatives in the decision-making process and to
obtain consent for these difficult processes.

Is Informed Consent Possible in the ICU?

It is obvious that there are certain obstacles for the process of consent in the
ICU setting. Given the limitations imposed by patient incapacity, the unpre-
dictability of critical illness, the often complex social situation of family
members, friends and partners seeking to represent the patient's wishes and
different national legislation, formal or informal consent must always be
obtained. This requires professional, empathic skills not ordinarily taught at
medical schools. Also, it is mandatory to create an open atmosphere in the
ICU, facilitating communication between the nursing staff and the relatives.
The decision-making process must be clearly documented for later analysis

and discussion, in order to improve future decisions. The issue of consent is complex and requires ethical skills as well as an empathic approach. This also involves sharing one's own attitudes and values. Be honest with your patients, their relatives, and the nursing staff! The main professional goal for all involved must be to avoid conflict over decisions concerning the care of the critically ill patient.

References

1. Ethells E, Shape C, Walsh P et al (1996) Bioethics for clinicians, 1: consent. CMAJ 155:177–180
2. Davis N, Pohlman A, Gehlbach B et al (2003) Improving the process of informed consent in the critically ill. JAMA 289:1963–1968
3. Fisher M (2004) Ethical issues in the intensive care unit. Curr Opin Crit Care 10:292–298
4. Manthous CA, DeGirolamo A, Haddad C et al (2003) Informed consent for medical procedures Local and national practices. Chest 124:1978–1984
5. Vincent J.-L. (1998) Information in the ICU: are we being honest with our patients? The results of a European questionnaire. Intensive Care Med 24:1251–1256
6. Sjökvist P, Berggren L, Svantesson M et al (1999) Withdrawal of life support—who should decide? Differences in attitudes among the general public, nurses and physicians. Intensive Care Med 25:949–954

Hepatorenal Syndrome

J. Besso, C. Pru, J. Padron, J. Plaz

Introduction

Initial reports by Frerichs (1861) and Flint (1863) [1], who had noted an association between advanced liver disease with ascites and acute oliguric renal
failure in the absence of significant histological changes in the kidneys, led
Heyd [2], and later Helwig and Schutz [3], to introduce the concept of the
hepatorenal syndrome (HRS) to explain the increased frequency of acute
renal failure after biliary surgery. However, because HRS could not be repro-
duced in animal models, pathophysiological concepts remained speculative
and its clinical entity was not generally accepted. During the 1950s, HRS was
more specifically characterised as a functional renal failure in patients with
advanced liver disease, electrolyte disturbances and low urinary sodium concentrations [4]. Hecker and Sherlock [5] showed its temporal reversibility by
norepinephrine administration. Over the next few decades, haemodynamic
and perfusion studies by Epstein and other investigators [6] identified
splanchnic and systemic vasodilatation and active renal vasoconstriction as
the pathophysiological hallmarks of HRS. Improved models of ascites and
circulatory dysfunction contributed to therapeutic advances, including the
introduction of large-volume paracentesis, vasopressin analogues, and transjugular intrahepatic stent-shunt (TIPS), which in turn have led to an
improved pathophysiological understanding of HRS [7].

Definition

HRS is defined as the development of renal failure in patients with severe
liver disease (acute or chronic) in the absence of any other identifiable cause
of renal pathology. It is diagnosed following the exclusion of other causes of
renal failure in patients with liver disease, such as hypovolaemia, drug

nephrotoxicity, sepsis or glomerulonephritis. A similar syndrome can also occur in the setting of acute liver failure [8].

In the kidney there is marked renal vasoconstriction, resulting in a low glomerular filtration rate (GFR). In the extrarenal circulation arterial vasodilatation predominates, resulting in reduction of the total systemic vascular resistance and arterial hypotension [9].

Diagnostic Criteria

The International Ascites Club (1996) group has defined the diagnostic criteria for HRS, and these are listed in Table 1 [8].

Table 1. International Ascites Club's criteria for diagnosis of hepatorenal syndrome

Major criteria	Chronic or acute liver disease with advanced hepatic failure and portal hypertension
	Low GFR, as indicated by serum creatinine > 1.5 mg/dl or 24-h creatinine clearance < 40 ml/min
	Absence of shock, ongoing bacterial infection, fluid loss, and current or recent treatment with nephrotoxic drugs
	Absence of gastrointestinal fluid losses (repeated vomiting or intense diarrhoea) or renal fluid losses (weight loss > 500 g/d for several days in patients with ascites without peripheral oedema or > 1000 ml in patients with peripheral oedema)
	No sustained improvement in renal function (decrease of serum creatinine to 1.5 mg/dl or less or increase in 24 h creatinine clearance to 40 ml/min or more) after withdrawal of diuretics and expansion of plasma volume with 1.5 l of isotonic saline
	Proteinuria < 500mg/d and no ultrasonographic evidence of obstructive uropathy or parenchymal renal disease
Additional criteria	Urine sodium < 10 meq/l
	Urine volume < 500 ml/d
	Urine osmolality > plasma osmolality
	Urine red blood cells < 50 per high-power field
	Serum sodium concentration < 130 meq/l

GFR, glomerular filtration rate

Two patterns of HRS are observed in clinical practice and have also been defined by the International Ascites Club [10]:

- Type 1 HRS is an acute form in which renal failure occurs spontaneously in patients with severe liver disease and is rapidly progressive. It is characterised by marked reduction of renal function, as defined by doubling of the initial serum creatinine to a level greater than 2.5 mg/dl, or a 50% reduction in initial 24-h creatinine clearance to < 20 ml/min within 2 weeks. Type 1 HRS has a poor prognosis, with 80% mortality at 2 weeks. Renal function can recover spontaneously following improvement in liver function. This is most frequently observed in acute liver failure or alcoholic hepatitis, or following acute decompensation against a background of cirrhosis. These patients are usually jaundiced and have significant coagulopathy. Death often results from a combination of hepatic and renal failure or from variceal bleeding.

- Type 2 HRS usually occurs in patients with diuretic resistance ascites. Renal failure has a slow course, with deterioration over months in some cases. It is also associated with a poor prognosis, although the survival time is longer than that of patients with type 1 HRS.

Application of these diagnostic criteria has become widely accepted as an important precondition of successful multicentre trials in HRS.

Use of the term 'pseudohepatorenal syndrome' to summarise other forms of renal failure in the setting of liver disease is not recommended [11].

Epidemiology

HRS occurs in about 4% of patients admitted to hospital with decompensated cirrhosis, the cumulative probability being 18% at 1 year, increasing to 39% at 5 years. Retrospective studies [12] indicate that HRS is present in approximately 17% of patients admitted to hospital with ascites and in more than 50% of cirrhotic patients dying of liver failure. The most frequent cause of renal failure in cirrhosis is spontaneous bacterial peritonitis (SBP). Approximately 30% of patients with SBP develop renal failure.

Type 1 HRS is characterised by rapid and progressive renal impairment and is precipitated most commonly by SBP. Type 1 HRS occurs in approximately 25% of patients with SBP, even when rapid resolution of the infection is obtained with antibiotics. Without treatment, the median survival of patients with HRS type 1 is less than 2 weeks, and virtually all patients die within 10 weeks after the onset of renal failure.

Type 2 HRS is characterised by a moderate and stable reduction in GFR and commonly occurs in patients with relatively well-preserved hepatic function. The median survival is 3–6 months. Although this is markedly longer than that in type 1 HRS, it is still shorter than that of patients with cirrhosis and ascites who do not have renal failure.

People of all races who have chronic liver disease are at risk of HRS, and its frequency is equal in both sexes; most patients with chronic liver disease are in the 4th–8th decade of life.

Prognosis

In a prospective study published by Gines et al., once HRS had developed the median survival was only 1.7 weeks, and it was poorer particularly in patients with apparent precipitating factors. Overall survival at 4 and 10 weeks was 20% and 10%, respectively. Patients with low urinary sodium excretion (< 5 meq/l) and reduced plasma osmolarity had a higher probability of developing HRS. Further risk factors for HRS development are presented in Table 2 [13, 14].

A recent prospective study [15] in 161 cirrhotic patients admitted to hospital with upper gastrointestinal bleeding confirmed that renal failure was still associated with elevated mortality: 55%, compared with 3% in patients without renal failure; although no differentiation was made between acute tubular necrosis and HRS, the development of nontransient renal failure was associated with an even poorer short-term prognosis (88% mortality).

Table 2. Risk factors for development of hepatorenal syndrome

Previous episodes of ascites
Absence of hepatomegaly
Poor nutritional status
Presence of oesophageal varices
Serum sodium < 133 mmol/l
Serum osmolality < 279 mosmol/l
Urine osmolality > 553 mosmol/l
Norepinephrine levels > 544pg/ml
Plasma renin activity > 3.5 ng /ml
Mean arterial pressure < 85 mmHg
GFR < 80 ml/min

GFR, glomerular filtration rate

Pathophysiology

The hallmark of HRS is renal vasoconstriction, although the pathogenesis is not fully understood. Multiple mechanisms are probably involved and include interplay between disturbances in systemic haemodynamics, activation of vasoconstrictor systems and a reduction in activity of the vasodilator systems [16–19]. The haemodynamic pattern of patients with HRS is characterised by increased cardiac output, low arterial pressure and reduced systemic vascular resistance. Renal vasoconstriction occurs in the absence of reduced cardiac output and blood volume, which is a point of contrast to most clinical conditions associated with renal hypoperfusion. Although the pattern of increased renal vascular resistance and decreased peripheral resistance is characteristic of HRS, it also occurs in other conditions, such as anaphylaxis and sepsis. Doppler studies of the brachial, middle cerebral and femoral arteries suggest that extrarenal resistance is increased in patients with HRS, while the splanchnic circulation is responsible for arterial vasodilatation and reduced total systemic vascular resistance.

The renin-angiotensin-aldosterone system (RAAS) and the sympathetic nervous system (SNS) are the predominant systems responsible for renal vasoconstriction [20]. The activity of both systems is increased in patients with cirrhosis and ascites, and this effect is magnified in HRS. In contrast, an inverse relationship exists between the activity of these two systems and renal plasma flow (RPF) and the glomerular filtration rate (GFR). Endothelin is another renal vasoconstrictor that is present in increased concentration in HRS, although its role in the pathogenesis of this syndrome has yet to be identified. Adenosine is well known for its vasodilator properties, although it acts as a vasoconstrictor in the lungs and kidneys. Elevated levels of adenosine are more common in patients with heightened activity of the RAAS and may work synergistically with angiotensin II to produce renal vasoconstriction in HRS. This effect has also been described with the powerful renal vasoconstrictor, leukotriene E4.

The vasoconstricting effect of these various systems is antagonised by local renal vasodilatory factors, the most important of which are the prostaglandins. Perhaps the strongest evidence supporting their role in renal perfusion is the marked decrease in RPF and the GFR when nonsteroidal medications known to bring about a sharp reduction in PG levels are administered.

Nitrous oxide (NO) is another vasodilator that is believed to play an important part in renal perfusion. Preliminary studies, predominantly based on animal experiments, have demonstrated that NO production is increased in the presence of cirrhosis, although NO inhibition does not result in renal vasoconstriction owing to a compensatory increase in PG synthesis. However, when both NO and PG production are inhibited, marked renal vasoconstriction develops.

These findings demonstrate that renal vasodilators have a critical role in maintaining renal perfusion, particularly in the presence of overactivity of renal vasoconstrictors. However, we do not yet know for certain whether vasoconstrictor activity becomes the predominant system in HRS and whether a reduction in the activity of the vasodilator system contributes to this [21–29].Various theories have been proposed to explain the development of HRS in cirrhosis. The two main ones are the arterial vasodilatation theory and the hepatorenal reflex theory. The first not only describes sodium and water retention in cirrhosis, but may also be the most rational hypothesis for the development of HRS. Splanchnic arteriolar vasodilatation in patients with compensated cirrhosis and portal hypertension may be mediated by several factors, the most important of which is probably NO. In the early phases of portal hypertension and compensated cirrhosis, this underfilling of the arterial bed causes a decrease in the effective arterial blood volume and results in homeostatic reflex activation of the endogenous vasoconstrictor systems. Activation of the RAAS and SNS occurs early with antidiuretic hormone secretion, a later event when a more marked derangement in circulatory function is present. This results in vasoconstriction not only of the renal vessels, but also in the vascular beds of the brain, muscle, spleen and extremities. The splanchnic circulation is resistant to these effects because of the continuous production of local vasodilators, such as NO. In the early phases of portal hypertension, renal perfusion is maintained within normal or near-normal limits as the vasodilatory systems antagonise the renal effects of the vasoconstrictor systems. However, as liver disease progress in severity, a critical level of vascular underfilling is achieved; renal vasodilatory systems are unable to counteract the maximal activation of the endogenous vasoconstrictors and/or intrarenal vasoconstrictors, which leads to uncontrolled renal vasoconstriction. Support for this hypothesis is provided by studies in which the administration of splanchnic vasoconstrictors in combination with volume expanders results in improvement in arterial pressure, RPF and GFR [30–34].

The alternative theory proposes that renal vasoconstriction in HRS is not related to systemic haemodynamics but is due either to a deficiency in the synthesis of a vasodilator factor or to a hepatorenal reflex that leads to renal vasoconstriction.

Evidence points to the vasodilatation theory as a more tangible explanation for the development of HRS.

Histopathology of HRS

In previous definitions of HRS, changes in renal histology were reported to be absent or minimal, which reflected a rapid progression to death after development of HRS. Considering that many patients with HRS currently receive aggressive supportive treatment including renal replacement therapy to prolong survival until liver transplantation, it seems obvious that prolonged renal hypoperfusion, renal medullary hypoxia and the high frequency of infectious complications ultimately contribute to histologically detectable renal damage. However, it is increasingly recognised that structural renal damage may already be found even before renal dysfunction becomes manifest. In a series of cirrhotic patients [35] undergoing liver transplantation, 100% of renal biopsies showed glomerular abnormalities. Tubular function is usually well preserved at the time when HRS develops, but tubular abnormalities, including increased B2 microglobulin excretion, have been reported in deeply jaundiced patients with HRS [36–38]. With progressive circulatory dysfunction, prolonged renal hypoperfusion may eventually result in acute tubular necrosis by increasing the susceptibility to additional insults by radiographic contrast agents, aminoglycosides, haemorrhage, endotoxinaemia or any other cause of medullary hypoxia. The presence of acute tubular necrosis could partially explain the slow or absent renal recovery in HRS type 1 even after the initiation of vasopressor support. For instance, a recent case study reports full recovery of renal function in dialysis-dependent HRS after 7 weeks of treatment with ornipressin, dopamine and intravenous albumin [39].

Prevention

The following measures may decrease the incidence of renal failure or HRS in patients with liver disease.

Prophylaxis Against Bacterial Infections

Bacterial infections occur in approximately 50% of patients with variceal haemorrhage, and antibiotic prophylaxis improves survival by approximately 10%. Patients who have had a previous episode of SBP have a 68% chance of recurrent infection at 1 year, and this carries a 33% chance of developing renal failure. As bacterial infections are an important cause of renal dysfunction in cirrhotic patients, prophylaxis with antibiotics is recommended in two clinical settings, namely variceal bleeding and a history of previous SBP [40, 41].

Volume Expansion

To prevent the development of renal failure in patients who develop SBP, it is now recommended that plasma volume expansion should be implemented in these patients by giving 20% albumin (1–1.5 g/kg over 1–3 days) at diagnosis to prevent circulatory dysfunction, renal impairment and mortality. Use of low-salt albumin as fluid replacement in patients undergoing large-volume paracentesis (8 g for each litre of ascitic fluid removed) is known to prevent paracentesis-induced circulatory dysfunction [42–45].

Judicious Use of Diuretics

It is important to identify the lowest effective dose of a diuretic for any individual patient, as diuretic-induced renal impairment is seen in approximately 20% of patients with ascites. It develops when the rate of diuresis exceeds the rate of ascites reabsorption, leading to intravascular volume depletion. Diuretic-induced renal impairment is usually moderate and rapidly reversible following diuretic withdrawal.

Avoidance of Nephrotoxic Drugs

Patients with cirrhosis and ascites are predisposed to the development of acute tubular necrosis during the use of aminoglycosides, with renal failure occurring in 33% of such patients as against 3–5% in the general population. Another important cause of renal failure is the use of nonsteroidal anti-inflammatory drugs (NSAIDs) [46].

Treatment

The ideal treatment for HRS is liver transplantation; however, because of the long waiting lists in the majority of transplant centres, most patient die before being offered a transplant. There is an urgent need for effective alternative therapies to increase survival chances for patients with HRS until transplantation can be performed. Treatment can be divided into initial management, pharmacological treatment and surgical manoeuvres.

Initial Management

Optimise fluid management. Renal function rarely recovers in the absence of liver recovery. The key goal in the management of these patients is to exclude reversible or treatable lesions (mainly hypovolaemia) and to support the patient until liver recovery or liver transplantation. The treatment of HRS is directed at reversing the haemodynamic changes induced by reduced renal perfusion pressure, stimulated sympathetic nervous system and increased synthesis of humoral and renal vasoconstrictor factors. In cirrhotic patients renal failure is frequently secondary to hypovolaemia (diuretics or gastrointestinal bleeding), NSAIDs or sepsis. Precipitating factors should be recognised and treated and nephrotoxic drugs, discontinued. All patients should be challenged with up 1.5 l of fluid, such as albumin solution or normal saline, to assess the renal response, as many patients with subclinical hypovolaemia will respond to this simple measure. This should be done with careful monitoring to avoid fluid overload. In practice, fluid overload is not usually a problem, as patients with severe liver disease function as 'fluid sumps' and their vasculature adapts to accommodate the extra fluid. This has been described by Hadengue et al., who reported increased venous compliance following fluid challenge in advanced cirrhosis [47, 48].

Monitor for sepsis. Evidence of sepsis should be sought in blood, ascitic, cannulae and urine cultures, and nonnephrotoxic broad-spectrum antibiotics should be started regardless of whether such evidence is found, as any delay in effective treatment of undiagnosed infection can increase mortality. In advanced cirrhosis, endotoxins and cytokines play important parts in fostering the hyperdynamic circulation and worsening renal function.

Optimise blood pressure. If mean arterial pressure is low (< 70 mmHg), it should be raised to approximately 85–90 mmHg or until urine output improves by infusing a vasopressor drug. Vasopressin, ornipressin, terlipressin, or noradrenaline infusion have all been used with some success. On physiological grounds it seems sensible to use either ornipressin or terlipressin as the first-line agent [49].

Paracentesis. Drainage of tense ascites may temporarily improve renal haemodynamics and renal function by decreasing renal venous pressure. There may be a modest fall in blood pressure following paracentesis. There is no evidence to support this approach, although it seems logical on the basis of published data. The fall in renal perfusion pressure due to decreased arterial pressure may of course counteract any beneficial effect and should therefore be counterbalanced by pressure support, as necessary [50].

Pharmacological Treatment

All the drugs that have been investigated in HRS have one overriding aim: to increase renal blood flow. This has been achieved either indirectly, by splanchnic vasoconstriction, or directly, using renal vasodilators. One of the principal difficulties has been the lack of agents that act purely on the splanchnic circulation. Drugs that 'spill over' into the systemic circulation may actually exacerbate the intense renal vasoconstriction already present. Currently, there is significant enthusiasm for the use of vasoconstrictor agents in HRS. However, the numbers of patients studied have been small, mortality remains high and there have been no randomised placebo-controlled trials. This deficit clearly needs to be addressed but the possibilities are limited by the relative rarity of patients with 'pure' HRS without such confounding variables as sepsis and gastrointestinal bleeding. Important aspect of the situation mentioned in these reports are the need for a pressor response to the agents used and the recurrence of abnormal renal function after the cessation of vasoconstrictor therapy. HRS is effectively a marker of poor hepatic function, and these agents are probably best utilised as a bridge to further improvement in liver function following either cessation of alcohol abuse or liver transplantation. Thus, the decision to use vasoconstrictor agents for HRS should be based on whether the patient is a realistic transplant candidate and, if not, whether liver function might improve. Patients who do not satisfy these criteria will be tested unnecessarily, merely prolonging the process of dying when palliative care would be more appropriate.

Dopamine. Nonpressor renal doses of dopamine [2–5 μg kg^{-1} min^{-1}) are frequently prescribed to patients with acute deterioration of renal function. As shown by a recent, large scale, randomised trial, early renal dose dopamine has no role in the prevention of acute renal failure in critically ill patients and does not significantly improve renal function in patients with HRS. At higher doses, dopamine worsens the hyperdynamic circulation by exaggerating splanchnic hyperaemia and increasing portal pressure and may cause tachyarrhythmia. Thus, the use of dopamine monotherapy seems to offer no benefit in HRS. Combination therapy with dopamine and vasopressors has produced inconsistent results in HRS. Because beneficial renal effects have been reported only with vasopressor, and not with dopamine, monotherapy, it seems unlikely that dopamine contributed to renal improvement in these studies [51–54].

Misoprostol. Misoprostol, a synthetic prostaglandin E-1 analogue, has been used to reverse renal vasoconstriction in HRS. Low doses of misoprostol are vasodilatory, natriuretic and diuretic, whereas high-dose misoprostol increases renal vascular tone and inhibits sodium and water excretion. None of the five studies investigating misoprostol in HRS seems to indicate substantial benefit. Improvement of renal function occurred in 1 of these studies, but could also be explained by volume expansion [55].

N-*Acetylcysteine.* In 1999, the group at the Royal Free Hospital reported their experience with *N*-acetylcysteine (NAC) for the treatment of HRS [56]. This was based on experimental models of acute cholestasis, in which the administration of NAC resulted in an improvement in renal function. Twelve patients with HRS were treated with intravenous NAC, without any adverse effects, and the survival rates were 67% and 58% at 1 month and 3 months, respectively (this included 2 patients who received liver transplantation after improvement in renal function). The mechanism of action remains unknown, but this interesting study encourages further optimism for medical treatment of a condition that once carried a hopeless diagnosis without liver transplantation. Controlled studies with longer follow-up may help answer these pressing questions.

Renal vasoconstrictor antagonists. Saralasin, an antagonist of angiotensin II receptors, was first used in 1979 in an attempt to reverse renal vasoconstriction. Because this drug inhibited the homeostatic response to hypotension commonly observed in patients with cirrhosis, it led to worsening hypotension and deterioration in renal function. Poor results were also observed with *phentolamine,* an alpha-adrenergic antagonist, highlighting the importance of the sympathetic nervous system in maintaining renal haemodynamics in patients with HRS.

Antagonists of endothelin A receptor. A recent case series by Soper et al. reported an improvement in GFR in patients with cirrhosis, ascites and HRS who received an endothelin A receptor antagonist. All patients showed a dose-dependent response in the form of improved inulin and para-aminohippurate excretion, RPF and GFR without changes in systemic haemodynamics. These patients were not candidates for liver transplantation and subsequently died. More work is needed to explore this therapeutic approach as a possible bridge to transplantation for patients with HRS [57-59].

Systemic vasoconstrictors. These medications have shown the most promise for treatment of HRS in recent years. Hecker and Sherlock used *norepinephrine* in 1956 to treat patients with cirrhosis who had HRS, and they were the first to describe an improvement in arterial pressure and urine output. However, no improvement was observed in the biochemical parameters of renal function, and all patients subsequently died.

Octapressin, a synthetic vasopressin analogue, was first used in 1970 to treat HRS type 1. RPF and the GFR improved in all patients, all of whom subsequently died of sepsis, gastrointestinal bleeding or liver failure. Because of these discouraging results, the use of alternative vasopressin analogues, particularly *ornipressin,* attracted attention. Two important studies by Lenz et al. [60, 61]

demonstrated that short term use of ornipressin resulted in an improvement in circulatory function and a significant increase in RPF and the GFR.

The *combination* of *ornipressin* and *albumin* was subsequently tried by Guevera in patients with HRS [49]. This idea was based on data suggesting that the combination of plasma volume expansion and vasoconstrictors nor-malised renal sodium and water handling in patients who had cirrhosis with ascites. In this study, 8 patients were originally treated for 15 days with orni-pressin and albumin. Treatment had to be discontinued in 4 patients after fewer than 9 days because of complications of ornipressin use that included ischaemic colitis, tongue ischaemia and glossitis. Although a marked improvement in the serum creatinine was observed during treatment, renal function deteriorated on treatment withdrawal. In the remaining 4 patients the improvement in RPF and the GFR was significant and was associated with a lowering of serum creatinine levels. These patients subsequently died, but no recurrence of HRS was observed. Owing to the high incidence of severe adverse effects with ornipressin, the same investigators used another vaso-pressin analogue with fewer adverse effects, namely *terlipressin*. In this study, nine patients were treated with *terlipressin* + *albumin* for 5-15 days. This treatment was associated with a marked fall in serum creatinine levels and an improvement in mean arterial pressure. Reversal of HRS was noted in seven of the nine patients, and HRS did not recur when treatment was discontinued. No adverse ischemic effects were reported: according to this study, *terli-pressin* with *albumin* is a safe and effective treatment for HRS [59-62].

Alpha adrenergic agonists. Angeli et al. showed that long-term administration of *midodrine* (an alpha-adrenergic agonist) and *octreotide* improved renal function in patients with HRS type 1 [65]. All patients also received *albumin*, and the results obtained with this approach were compared against those observed with dopamine at nonpressor doses. None of the patients treated with dopamine showed any improvement in renal function, but in all the patients treated with midodrine, octreotide and volume expansion renal function did improve. No adverse effects were reported in these patients. Gulberg et al. treated seven patients who had cirrhosis and HRS type 1 with a combination of ornipressin and dopamine for infusion periods as long as 27 days, but only three of the seven patients survived [62]. This treatment can be used as a bridge to liver transplantation [61, 65].

Aquaretic agents. K-Opioid antagonists inhibit antidiuretic hormone secretion by the neurohypophysis and induce water excretion. Administration of *niravo-line* at doses ranging from 0.5 to 2 mg induced a strong aquaretic response and was well tolerated in 18 cirrhotic patients with preserved renal function, but no data are available on the use of niravoline in patients with HRS.

Surgical Manoeuvres

Transjugular intrahepatic portosystemic shunting. It is well documented that portal hypertension plays a central role in the development of refractory ascites and HRS. Earlier studies showed improved renal function after side-to-side portocaval shunting, but at the cost of a high surgical mortality in advanced cirrhosis. The transjugular intrahepatic portosystemic shunt (TIPS) was introduced as a less invasive method of reducing increased portal pressure. Guevarra et al. have investigated hepatic and renal haemodynamic changes after placement of TIPS in patients with HRS. One month after placement of TIPS a marked improvement in renal function was observed, as indicated by a significant reduction in serum creatinine and blood urea nitrogen and increased urine volume, RPF and GFR. These improvements were associated with a reduction in plasma rennin, aldosterone and norepinephrine activity. These changes were statistically significant, albeit less pronounced than observed in a similar group of patients receiving ornipressin and albumin infusions. Renal improvements were more pronounced at 30 days than at 7 days, possibly because of the deleterious effects of contrast media or the resolution of concomitant problems. After TIPS, GFR improved significantly but did not reach normal values, suggesting that TIPS does not correct all mechanisms contributing to HRS. Brensing et al. [65] found a sustained improvement of renal function after TIPS in 31 patients with type 1 or 2 HRS, allowing the discontinuation of haemodialysis in four of seven patients. After TIPS 3-, 6-, 12- and 18-month survival rates were 81%, 71%, 48% and 35%, respectively, in the total patient cohort, with survival in HRS type 1 patients being significantly worse than in the others. The use of TIPS to prolong survival until liver transplantation seems promising [65-68].

Other surgical shunts. Despite the theoretical benefit of improving portal hypertension and thus HRS by means of a portosystemic shunt, only a few scattered case reports have shown any benefit. Currently, particularly with the recent introduction of TIPS, portocaval shunts are not indicated in this setting.

Renal replacement therapy. Many clinicians are reluctant to institute renal replacement therapy in advanced cirrhosis, because the outcome is poor unless liver transplantation is a realistic option. Intermittent haemodialysis can be a problem because patients with HRS are prone to develop circulatory and coagulation problems, and biocompatibility is also a problematic issue [69]. In an early study in the United Kingdom 100% mortality was observed in cirrhotic patients with HRS despite early institution of renal support [70]. However, modern renal replacement therapies such as continuous endogenous haemofiltration (CVVH) are certainly capable of prolonging life in patients with type 1 HRS who have not responded to medical therapies or TIPS. Because the underlying hepatic problem persists, the long-term prognosis is grim and treatment should be confined to patients who are candidates for liver transplantation or have a realistic chance of hepatic recovery. The molecular adsorbent recirculating system (MARS) is a modified dialysis method that uses albumin-containing dialysate in a closed-loop secondary circuit for adsorptive removal of albumin-bound toxins. In a randomised study, short-term survival of eight HRS patients treated with MARS was superior to that of five other HRS patients treated with CVVH [71]. In contrast to previous reports on haemodialysis, treatment was well tolerated. Unfortunately, the study was terminated after enrolment of only 13 patients, which makes evaluation of any influence on mortality difficult. Moreover, the control group seems to have received a smaller dialytic dose: creatinine levels were decreased in the MARS group only. Nonetheless, the favourable effects of this system deserve evaluation in a prospective study of adequate power.

Liver transplantation. Liver transplantation is the ideal treatment for HRS, but is completely dependent on the availability of Donors. Patients with HRS have a higher risk of postoperative morbidity, early mortality and longer hospitalisation than other transplant recipients. Gonwa et al. [72] reported that at least one third of such patients require haemodialysis postoperatively, with a smaller proportion (5%) requiring long-term dialysis. Because renal dysfunction is common in the first few days after transplantation, avoidance nephrotoxic immunosuppressants is generally recommended until renal function is recovered. However, the GFR gradually improves to an average of 40–50 ml/min by the 6th postoperative week. The systemic and neurohumoral abnormalities associated with HRS also resolve in the 1st postoperative month. Long-term survival rates are excellent, with the survival rate at 3 years approaching approximately 60%. This is only slightly lower than the 70–80% survival rate of transplant recipients without HRS and is markedly better than the survival rate of patients with HRS who do not receive transplants, which is virtually nil at 3 years [73, 74].

References

1. Flint A (1863) Clinical report on hydro-peritoneum, based on analysis of forty-six cases. Am J Med Sci 45:306–339
2. Heyd CG (1924) The liver and its relation to chronic abdominal infection. Ann Surg 79:55–77
3. Helwig FC, Schutz CB (1932) A liver-kidney syndrome: Clinical, pathologic and experimental studies. Surg Gynecol Obstet 55:570–580
4. Papper S, Belsky JL, Bleifer KH (1932) Renal failure in Laennec's cirrhosis of the liver. I. Clinical and laboratory features. Ann Intern Med 57:759–773

5. Hecker R, Sherlock S (1956) Electrolyte and circulatory changes in terminal liver failure. Lancet 2:1121–1125
6. Epstein M, Berk DP, Hollenberg NK et al (1970) Renal failure in the patient with cirrhosis. The role of active vasoconstriction. Am J Med 49:175–185
7. Arroyo V, Bataller R (1999) Historical notes on ascites in cirrhosis. In: Arroyo V, Gines P, Rodes J et al (eds) Ascites and renal dysfunction in liver disease. Blackwell Science, Oxford, pp 3–13
8. Arroyo V, Gines P, Gerbes AL et al (1996) Definition and diagnostic criteria of refractory ascites and hepatorenal syndrome in cirrhosis. Hepatology 23:164–176
9. Arroyo V, Gines P, Jimenez V et al (1999) Renal dysfunction in cirrhosis. In: Bircher J, Benhamou J-P, McIntyre N et al (eds) Oxford textbook of clinical hepatology. Oxford University Press, Oxford, pp 733–761
10. Arroyo V, Gines P, Gerbes AL et al (1996) Definition and diagnostic criteria of refractory ascites and hepatorenal syndrome in cirrhosis. International Ascites Club Hepatology 23:164–176
11. Conn HO (1973) A rational approach to the hepatorenal syndrome. Gastroenterology 65:321–340
12. Gines A, Escorsell A, Gines P et al (1993) Incidence, predictive factors, and prognosis of the hepatorenal syndrome in cirrhosis with ascites. Gastroenterology 105:229–236
13. Gines P, Martin P-Y, Niederberger M (1997) Prognostic significance of renal dysfunction in cirrhosis. Kidney Int Suppl 51:S77–S82
14. Kramer L, Horl WH (2002) Hepatorenal syndrome. Semin Nephrol 22:290–301
15. Hampel H, Bynum GD, Zamora E et al (2001) Risk factors for the development of renal dysfunction in hospitalized patients with cirrhosis. Am J Gastroenterol 96:2206–2210
16. Cardenas A, Gines P, Uriz J et al (2001) Renal failure after upper gastrointestinal bleeding in cirrhosis: incidence, clinical course, predictive factors, and short-term prognosis. Hepatology 34:671–676
17. Schrier RW, Arroyo V, Bernardi M et al (1988) Peripheral arterial vasodilation hypothesis: a proposal for the initiation of renal sodium and water retention in cirrhosis. Hepatology 8:1151–1157
18. Fernandez-Seara J, Prieto J, Quiroga J et al (1989) Systemic and regional hemodynamics in patients with liver cirrhosis and ascites with and without functional renal failure. Gastroenterology 97:1304–1312
19. Koyama S, Kanai K, Aibiki M et al (1988) Reflex increase in renal nerve activity during acutely altered portal venous pressure. J Auton Nerv Syst 23:55–62
20. Ming Z, Smyth DD, Lautt WW (2002) Decreases in portal flow trigger a hepatorenal reflex to inhibit renal sodium and water excretion in rats: role of adenosine. Hepatology 35:167–175
21. Arroyo V, Bosch J, Rivera F et al (1979) The renin angiotensin system in cirrhosis. Its relation to functional renal failure. In: Bartoli E, Chiandussi L (eds) Hepatorenal syndrome. Piccin Medical Books, Padua, pp 201–29
22. Schriern RW, Arroyo V, Bernardi M et al (1988) Peripheral arterial vasodilation hypothesis: a proposal for the initiation of renal sodium and water retention in cirrhosis. Hepatology 8:1151–1157
23. Colle I, Moreau R, Pessione F et al (2001) Relationship between haemodynamic alterations and the development of ascites or refractory ascites in patients with cirrhosis. Eur J Gastroenterol Hepatol 13:251–256
24. Platt JF, Ellis JH, Rubin JM et al (1994) Renal duplex Doppler ultrasonography: a non

invasive predictor of kidney dysfunction and hepatorenal failure in liver disease. Hepatology 20:362–369

25. Epstein M (1986) Renal prostaglandins and the control of renal function in liver disease. Am J Med 80:46–55

26. Vallance P, Moncada S (1991) Hyperdynamic circulation in cirrhosis: a role for nitric oxide? Lancet 337:776–778

27. Sogni P, Garnier P, Gadano A et al (1995) Endogenous pulmonary nitric oxide production measured from exhaled air is increased in patients with severe cirrhosis. J Hepatol 23:471–473

28. Moncada S, Higgs A (1991) The L-arginine-nitric oxide pathway. N Engl J Med 329:2002–2012

29. Genesca J, Gonzalez A, Segura R et al (1999) Interleukin-6, nitric oxide, and the clinical and hemodynamic alterations of patients with liver cirrhosis. Am J Gastroenterol 94:169–177

30. Pateron D, Tazi KA, Sogni P et al (2000) Role of aortic nitric oxide synthase in the systemic vasodilation of portal hypertension. Gastroenterology 119:196–200

31. Rockey DC, Chung JJ (1998) Reduced nitric oxide production by endothelial cells in cirrhotic rat liver: endothelial dysfunction in portal hypertension. Gastroenterology 114:344–351

32. Song D, Liu H, Sharkey KA et al (2002) Hyperdynamic circulation in portal-hypertensive rats is dependent on central c-fos gene expression. Hepatology 35:159–166

33. Gadano A, Moreau R, Heller J et al (1999) Relation between severity of liver disease and renal oxygen consumption in patients with cirrhosis. Gut 45:117–121

34. Helmy A, Jalan R, Newby DE et al (2000) Role of angiotensin II in regulation of basal and sympathetically stimulated vascular tone in early and advanced cirrhosis. Gastroenterology 118:565–572

35. Gerbes AL, Gülberg V, Bilzer M (1998) Endothelin and other mediators in the pathophysiology of portal hypertension. Digestion 59 [Suppl 2]:8–10

36. Lhotta K (2002) Beyond hepatorenal syndrome-glomerulonephritis in patients with liver disease. Semin Nephrol 22:302–308

37. Rector WG Jr, Kanel GC, Rakela J et al (1985) Tubular dysfunction in the deeply jaundiced patient with hepatorenal syndrome. Hepatology 5:321–326

38. Heyman SN, Darmon D, Goldfarb M et al (2000) Endotoxin-induced renal failure. I. A role for altered renal microcirculation. Exp Nephrol 8:266–274

39. Mandal AK, Lansing M, Fahmy A (1982) Acute tubular necrosis in hepatorenal syndrome: an electron microscopy study. Am J Kidney Dis 2:363–374

40. Eckardt KU, Frei U (2000) Reversibility of hepatorenal syndrome in an anuric patient with Child C cirrhosis requiring haemodialysis for 7 weeks. Nephrol Dial Transplant 15:1063–1065

41. Gines P, Rimola A, Planas R et al (1990) Norfloxacin prevents spontaneous bacterial peritonitis recurrence in cirrhosis: results of a double blind, placebo-controlled trial. Hepatology 12:716–724

42. Follo A, Llovet JM, Navasa M et al (1994) Renal impairment after spontaneous bacterial peritonitis in cirrhosis: predictive factors of infection resolution and survival in patients with cefotaxime. Hepatology 20:1495–1501

43. Sort P, Navasa M, Arroyo V et al (1999) Effect of intravenous albumin on renal impairment and mortality in patients with cirrhosis and spontaneous bacterial peritonitis. N Engl J Med 341:403–409

44. Gines P, Tito L, Arroyo V et al (1988) Randomized comparative study of therapeutic paracentesis with and without intravenous albumin in cirrhosis. Gastroenterology 84:1493–1502

45. Gines P, Fernandez-Esparrach G, Monescillo A et al (1996) Randomized trial comparing albumin, dextran 70, and polygeline in cirrhotic patients with ascites treated by paracentesis. Gastroenterology 111:1002–1010

46. Gines P, Arroyo V (2000) Is there still a need for albumin infusions to treat patients with liver disease? Gut 46:588–590

47. Cabrera J, Arroyo V, Ballesta AM et al (1982) Aminoglycoside toxicity in cirrhosis. Value of urinary beta-2 microglobulin to discriminate functional renal failure from acute tubular damage. Gastroenterology 82:97–105

48. Hadengue A, Moreau R, Gaudin C et al (1992) Total effective vascular compliance in patients with cirrhosis: a study of the response to acute blood volume expansion. Hepatology 15:809–815

49. Guevara M, Gines P, Fernandez-Esparrach G et al (1998) Reversibility of hepatorenal syndrome by prolonged administration of ornipressin and plasma volume expansion. Hepatology 27:35–41

50. Uriz J, Cardenas A, Sort P et al (2000) Telipressin plus albumin infusion: an effective and safe therapy of hepatorenal syndrome. J Hepatol 33:43–48

51. Gentilini P (1999) Hepatorenal syndrome and ascites -an introduction. Liver 19 [Suppl]:5–14

52. Bacq Y, Gaudin C, Hadengue A et al (1991) Systemic, splanchnic and renal hemodynamic effects of a dopaminergic dose of dopamine in patients with cirrhosis. Hepatology 14:483–487

53. Barnardo DE, Baldus WP, Maher FT (1970) Effects of dopamine on renal function in patients with cirrhosis. Gastroenterology 58:524–531

54. Bellomo R, Chapman M, Finfer S et al (2000) Low-dose dopamine in patients with early renal dysfunction: a placebo–controlled randomised trial. Australian and New Zealand Intensive Care Society (ANZICS) Clinical Trials Group. Lancet 356:2139–2143

55. Dagher L, Patch D, Marley R et al (2000) Pharmacological treatment of the hepatorenal syndrome in cirrhotic patients (review article). Aliment Pharmacol Ther 14:515–521

56. Fevery J, Van Cutsem E, Nevens F et al (1990) Reversal of hepatorenal syndrome in four patients by peroral misoprostol (prostaglandin E1 analogue) and albumin administration. J Hepatol 11:153–158

57. Holt S, Marley R, Fernando B et al (1999) Improvement of renal function in hepatorenal syndrome with N-acetyl cysteine. Lancet 353:294

58. Moore K, Wendon J, Frazer M et al (1992) Plasma endothelin immunoreactivity in liver disease and the hepatorenal syndrome. N Engl J Med 327:1774–1778

59. Soper CP, Latif AB, Bending MR (1996) Amelioration of hepatorenal syndrome with selective endothelin-A antagonist. Lancet 347:1842–1843

60. Lenz K, Hornatgl H, Druml W et al (1989) Beneficial effect of 8-ornithine vasopressin on renal dysfunction in decompensated cirrhosis. Gut 30:90–96

61. Lenz K, Druml W, Kleinberger G et al (1985) Enhancement of renal function with ornipressin in a patient with decompensated cirrhosis. Gut 26:1385–1386

62. Gulberg V, Bilzer M, Gerbes AL (1999) Long-term therapy and retreatment of hepatorenal syndrome type 1 with omipressin and dopamine. Hepatology 30:870–875

63. Hadengue A, Gadano A, Moreau R et al (1998) Beneficial effects of the 2-day administration of terlipressin in patients with cirrhosis and hepatorenal syndrome. J Hepatol 29:565–570

64. Kaffy F, Borderie C, Chagneau C et al (1999) Octreotide in the treatment of the hepatorenal syndrome in cirrhotic patients. J Hepatol 30:174

65. Angeli P, Volpin R, Gerunda G et al (1999) Reversal of type 1 hepatorenal syndrome with the administration of midodrine and octreotide. Hepatology 29:1690–1697

66. Rösch J, Keller FS (2001) Transjugular intrahepatic portosystemic shunt: Present status, comparison with endoscopic therapy and shunt surgery, and future perspectives. World J Surg 25:337–345

67. Rössle M, Haag K, Ochs A et al (1994) The transjugular intrahepatic portosystemic stent-shunt procedure for variceal bleeding. N Engl J Med 330:165–171

68. Brensing KA, Textor J, Perz J et al (2000) Long term outcome after transjugular intrahepatic portosystemic stent-shunt in non transplant cirrhotics with hepatorenal syndrome: a phase II study. Gut 47:288–295

69. Colombato LA, Spahr L, Martinet JP et al (1996) Haemodynamic adaptation two months after transjugular intrahepatic portosystemic shunt (TPS) in cirrhotic patients. Gut 39:600–604

70. Kramer L, Gendo A, Madl C et al (2000) Biocompatibility of a cuprophane charcoal-based detoxification device in cirrhotic patients with hepatic encephalopathy. Am J Kidney Dis 36:1193–1200

71. Wilkinson SP, Weston MJ, Parsons V et al (1977) Dialysis in the treatment of renal failure in patients with liver disease. Clin Nephrol 8:287–292

72. Mitzner SR, Stange J, Klammt S et al (2000) Improvement of hepatorenal syndrome with extracorporeal albumin dialysis MARS: result of a prospective, randomized, controlled clinical trial. Liver Transplant 6:277–286

73. Gonwa TA, Klintmalm GB, Levy M et al (1995) Impact of pretransplant renal function on survival after liver transplantation. Transplantation 59:361–365

74. Gonwa TA, Mai ML, Melton LB et al (2001) End-stage renal disease (ESRD) after orthotopic liver transplantation (OLTX) using calcineurin-based immunotherapy: risk of development and treatment. Transplantation 72:1934–1939

HIV/AIDS in Developing Countries

S. Bhagwanjee

Background

The HIV/AIDS epidemic in developing countries has raised unique challenges. Total health care expenditure is low in comparison to developed countries. The overwhelming effect of infectious diseases, malnutrition, and inadequate education, singularly and in combination seriously limit the capacity of such countries to deal with HIV/AIDS with effective long-term strategies. This review will focus on three aspects of the epidemic with emphasis on their impact on critically ill patients in developing countries.

The overall prevalence of HIV infection varies from 5-20% depending on the age group, stage of the epidemic, and relative efficiency of prevention strategies [1]. Nevertheless, for various reasons, the proportion of patients that reach intensive care units (ICUs) is relatively small. Careful consideration is needed in clinical decision making in dealing with these patients. Major ethical dilemmas are raised around issues of resource allocation, informed consent and disclosure of HIV status. Lastly, some attention will be paid to the question of protection for health care workers.

Clinical Aspects

Early in the epidemic, many clinicians believed that the outcome from clinical therapy was poor in patients who were HIV positive. Such perceptions were subjective and were significantly influenced by the lack of data. As a consequence, many practices were driven toward limiting care offered to HIV positive patients. Available data from developed countries were not readily translatable into practice in developing countries because the clinical scenarios were not comparable [2]. A large randomised, double blind study conducted in South Africa compared the outcome of patients who were incidentally HIV positive to HIV negative patients and found no difference in outcome when these patients were admitted to ICU for diseases unrelated to their HIV status [3]. Such data changed the attitude to this patient population. Equally there emerged clear data demonstrating a poor outcome in severely immuno-compromised children admitted to ICU for HIV related complications [4]. The introduction of highly active anti-retroviral therapy as the standard of care in many emerging countries has also impacted on clinical outcome [5] (by augmenting immune function) such that it is ethically unacceptable to deny patients who are incidentally HIV positive intensive care. The commonest reason for ICU admission is respiratory tract sepsis. The spectrum of disease in such patients is indicated in Table 1. As opposed to developed countries, community acquired pneumonia and tuberculosis are the leading causes of respiratory tract sepsis in developing countries. Therapy must therefore be directed toward these causative organisms.

Table 1.

Developed countries	Developing countries
PCP	CAP
CMV	TB
TB	Mixed
Other	PCP

Thoracic complications that require surgical intervention are usually necessary for diagnostic purposes and to manage complications of respiratory tract sepsis. In this situation, aggressive surgery has been shown to be effective [6].

Informed Consent in the Critically Ill HIV Positive Patient

Written informed consent is the standard of care for medical and surgical treatment of all patients. Furthermore, indiscriminate disclosure of HIV status is unacceptable particularly given the social stigma attached to being HIV positive. Lastly, it is accepted practice that decisions regarding the withholding and withdrawal of therapy must be based on the best available evidence. These considerations are particularly difficult in the setting of HIV/AIDS as illustrated by the cases below. All considerations must be based on assessments of the benefit to the patient, family, health care workers, and society.

Consent for Testing

While it is common practice for patients to be tested routinely prior to surgery in some institutions, there is no evidence that this practice is beneficial. The high overall prevalence of HIV/AIDS has entrenched routine application of universal precautions for the protection of health care workers and other patients. Testing for HIV is appropriate when exposure is suspected or when patients present with HIV related complications. Testing will influence patient management. In this situation pre and post test counselling by trained personnel is mandatory. Current guidelines and legislation prohibit the conduct of HIV testing without prior informed consent. There are, however, situations where clinicians have presented cogent arguments for the conduct of HIV tests without consent. The following clinical scenarios demonstrate some of the issues.

Case 1

A clinician conducting general anaesthesia for surgery suffers an accidental needle-stick injury during surgery. It has been established that prophylactic anti-retroviral (ARV) therapy in this situation must be administered as early as possible (preferably within 30 minutes) to limit the risk to the health care worker. HIV testing of the patient should be conducted without consent and pre and post test counselling should be performed as soon as it is feasible after surgery. If the test result is not be available within this time (for logistic reasons), then it is advisable to commence prophylactic ARV therapy and to continue until the result is available. It is also essential that disclosure of the patients' HIV status is limited to the primary physician (who will then advise the patient about appropriate care), the injured health care worker, and the doctor caring for the health care worker.

Case 2

A 25-year-old patient presents with community-acquired pneumonia. Empiric treatment is commenced and bacteriology results suggest that the correct therapy has been instituted based on culture and susceptibility testing. Forty eight hours later, the patient deteriorates and develops signs of peritonism. Chest X-ray demonstrates progression of the pneumonia (despite appropriate therapy) and the patient now requires ventilation for respiratory failure. At this point the following should be considered:
1. The initial bacteriological diagnosis and therefore therapy was incorrect
2. Multiple pathogens are responsible for the pneumonia
3. The patient has atypical pneumonia
4. The patient is immunocompromised and atypical co-infections must be considered.

If 1 and 2 are unlikely or excluded, most clinicians would resort to an HIV test. Current legislation suggests that the patient should be treated as though he/she is HIV positive and testing should only be performed after the patient has recovered and can consent to testing. This approach is unacceptable for several reasons. Firstly, the common diagnosis to entertain if the patient was HIV positive would be tuberculosis. This necessitates polypharmacy that takes several days even weeks before clinical response can be expected. If the patient was not negative this would result in inappropriate management and unreasonable expectations. Secondly, the patient would be denied a laparotomy in the initial stages since the treatment of GI tract tuberculosis is medical. This would be totally inappropriate in the presence of bacterial pneumonia. Thirdly, co-infection with other bacterial pathogens is common in HIV and empiric therapy for these organisms would be considered mandatory by many clinicians. Fourthly, if the patient were HIV negative treatment for atypical pneumonia and laparotomy would be mandatory.

Disclosure of HIV Results

Disclosure of a patients' HIV status to a colleague or relative is unacceptable except under exceptional circumstances. The following cases are illustrative.

Case 3

A 39-year-old, known HIV positive male patient dies from disseminated tuberculosis. The family is clearly at risk, having been exposed to tuberculosis. Disclosure of this exposure and screening of the family is appropriate. If sexually active, the wife is at risk with respect to HIV. In this situation, the wife should be counselled regarding the HIV risk, the need for testing and the potential for ARV therapy in the event she is positive. If, on the other hand, the patient was not sexually active (or unmarried), there is no risk of HIV exposure to the family and therefore disclosure of HIV status of the patient would be inappropriate.

If the same patient was to survive his illness, he should be counselled regarding exposure of the family to tuberculosis and the wife to HIV. If, despite adequate counselling, the patient refuses to discuss this with his wife, it is reasonable to disclose his status and hence the risk with the wife.

Case 4

A 26-year-old patient known to be HIV positive is referred for open reduction and internal fixation of a femur fracture. In this situation the surgeon should inform the anaesthesiologist about the HIV status since it is likely to affect patient management. The patient is at increased risk for deep venous thrombosis (DVT) and post-operative sepsis. Anaesthetic management should be tailored to deal with these potential complications.

Since universal precautions are applied at all times, potential exposure to health care workers does not justify disclosure of HIV status.

Withholding and Withdrawing Treatment

Decisions regarding the withholding and withdrawing of treatment are perhaps the most controversial aspect of dealing with HIV/AIDS. In this regard, it is essential that all decisions regarding patient care be determined by objective evidence. It is current practice in some units for HIV testing to be routinely performed on all patients needing certain types of surgery e.g. cardiac surgery. In this situation it has been argued that the allocation of a scarce resource to a patient with a diminished life span is inappropriate. Where ARV therapy is routinely available such arguments are inappropriate. In South Africa ARV therapy is currently available to prevent maternal-foetal transmission. The introduction of ARV therapy to all HIV positive patients was recently endorsed by cabinet, a decision that will change the spectrum of HIV/AIDS in South Africa. Careful consideration of these factors, the extent of HIV progression and the risks posed by surgery must be the basis for such decisions.

By the same token, the withdrawal of treatment must be guided in the first instance by the test of futility. Futility implies sufficient evidence that treatment will not improve quality and/or quantity of life.

Case 5

A 48-year-old HIV positive patient with pulmonary tuberculosis, wasting, and oral candidiasis is referred for repair of an abdominal aortic aneurysm. The surgeon books the patient for elective surgery. This patient has AIDS with a poor 6 month survival from the advanced state of HIV infection. This assessment can be objectively validated by a low CD4 count (likely to be < 200). A high viral load will typically co-exist in this situation and is not essential for the decision. Surgical intervention in this situation is futile; the patient should therefore not be offered surgery. Therapy is therefore withheld.

Case 6

A 12-year-old HIV positive child with typhoid perforation of the small bowel is referred for laparotomy. Leucopaenia and a CD4 count of 300 are documented prior to surgery. Surgery proceeds uneventfully, with repairs being effected in the small bowel. Two days post-operatively the child develops respiratory failure, leucopaenia persists, CD4 count drops to 120 and renal failure. These complications persist despite treatment for four days at which point ultrasound identifies intra-abdominal abscess. The patient is then presented for repeat laparotomy. At this point further intervention is futile since the mortality is > 95% regardless of HIV status. The fact that the patient is a child should not influence the decision to withdraw treatment at this time.

Protection of Health Care Workers

The high prevalence of HIV worldwide has prompted the implementation of universal precautions [7]. Whilst financial and practical issues limit the potential for implementation of such strategies (a discussion of which is beyond the scope of this paper), there is abundant evidence indicating the need for education amongst health care workers in this regard [8]. Although hepatitis is a more commonly acquired occupational disease, HIV provokes greater fear among most health care workers. The risk of HIV transmission from needle-stick injuries and blood splashes is estimated to about 0.5% [7]. Several factors influence the risk of a single exposure. High risk factors include: hollow needles (compared to solid needles), depth of injection, viral load of the patient, extent of ARV therapy in the patient and time to ingestion of appropriate prophylactic treatment. The key to a successful preventive strategy rests in effective policy making followed by an active educational program. In our institution exposure is categorised as high or low risk based on the factors mentioned above. A high risk exposure is identified early such that prophylaxis maybe implemented within thirty minutes. The system is designed in such a way that an infectious disease physician is available to assist 24 hours a day to assist with identification of high risk exposures and that prophylactic drugs are available from high activity areas (casualty, operating rooms and ICUs).

Equally, efforts are in place to ensure effective preventive strategies. For example, delivery systems for intravenous fluids routinely include 'needleless' ports which preclude the use of needles for intravenous drug or blood administration. Notwithstanding such steps, errors in practice continue to occur. In parallel with practices elsewhere, steps have been implemented to limit the use of blood and blood products to minimise the exposure of patients and staff to donor contaminated blood.

Conclusions

The HIV/AIDS epidemic represents one of the greatest clinical challenges with the addition of unique circumstances in the developing world. The poor correlation of clinical patterns between developed and developing countries demands that we constantly validate clinical practice based on objective published data from studies conducted in the developing world.

The unique ethical issues posed by HIV further challenge the clinician to make careful ethical decisions based on the reality of conditions in each individual situation.

Lastly, every effort must be made to ensure the safety of the health care worker via the adoption of appropriate preventive and prophylactic protocols. This in conjunction with an effective ongoing educational program is crucial for the preservation of a healthy and motivated health care work force.

References

1. Connolly C, Shisana O, Colvin M et al (2004) Epidemiology of HIV in South Africa—results of a national, community-based survey. S Afr Med J 94(9):776–781
2. Gilks CF (1993) The clinical challenge of the HIV epidemic in the developing world. Lancet 342:1037–1039
3. Bhagwanjee S, Muckart DJJ, Jeena PM et al (1997) HIV status does not influence the outcome of patients admitted to a Surgical Intensive Care Unit. Br Med J 314:1077–1081
4. Jeena PM, Coovadia HM, Bhagwanjee S (1996) Prospective, controlled study of the outcome of human immunodeficiency virus-1 antibody-positive children admitted to an intensive care unit. Crit Care Med 24:963–967
5. Narasimhan M, Posner AJ, DePalo VA et al (2004) Intensive care in patients with HIV infection in the era of highly active antiretroviral therapy. Chest 125:1800–1804
6. DiMaio JM, Wait MA (1999) The thoracic surgeon's role in the management of patients with HIV infection and AIDS. Chest Surg Clin N Am 9:97–111
7. Ippolito G, Puro V, Heptonstall J et al (1999) Occupational human immunodeficiency virus infection in health care workers: worldwide cases through September. Clin Infect Dis 28:365–383
8. DeJoy DM, Gershon RR, Murphy LR et al (1996) A work-systems analysis of compliance with universal precautions among health care workers. Health Educ Q 23:159–174

Do Not Attempt Resuscitation Order

F.J. DE LATORRE

Since 1974, when the first policies about 'do not attempt resuscitation' orders were published [1], the decision not to resuscitate patients in cardiac arrest has been a controversial issue in medical practice. For this reason, the 'do not attempt resuscitation' order is, perhaps, the directive and the decision to withhold medical treatment with the widest bibliography. In this review, in accordance with the 2000 Guidelines for Cardiopulmonary Resuscitation [2], I will use the term 'do not attempt resuscitation (DNAR)' instead of the more popular 'do not resuscitate (DNR)'. The first sentence indicates more clearly the decision to take, because the success of a resuscitation is not always guaranteed.

In the practice of resuscitation, it has been accepted for many years that when a person has suffered a sudden cardiac arrest, resuscitation manoeuvres should always be started 'except in narrowly defined circumstances' [3]. This concept has not changed in the current guidelines [2, 4]. This concept is unique in the practice of medicine, and it is based on the facts that it is an emergency and also a benefit for the patient [5]. The rationale lies in the belief that life is precious and that resuscitation will be successful. However, the latter is not true and the rate of survival ranges between 15-25% [6] and many of the initially resuscitated patients have residual impairment if the resuscitation is not completely achieved [7], thus prolonging the suffering of both patients and relatives [8]. Today we know well that all attempts at resuscitation should be previously assessed and agreed with the patient or relative, if this is possible [9].

What Are the Real Possibilities of Success in Resuscitation?

The rationale for always starting cardiopulmonary resuscitation (CPR) manoeuvres in a cardiac arrest in patients without a poor prognosis due to underlying diseases is based on the good results in many individual patients, with both good neurological recovery and quality of life. However, the rate of survival after a cardiac arrest has been not higher than 25% in the better results [10] and the average standard rate is 6% of survivors emerging from an out-of-hospital cardiac arrest [11] and it may be as lower as 1.4% in New York City [12]. In hospital cardiac arrests the current survival after resuscitation to hospital discharge is 17% in the USA, according to the National Registry of Cardiopulmonary Resuscitation [13].

In recent years, an improvement in positive outcome after cardiac arrest has been observed in some special sites, as in the casinos of Las Vegas, with the use of automated external defibrillators by trained non-healthcare personnel, with a 53% of survival to discharge from the hospital [14]. A significant increase in survival has been observed in the PAD Trial [15] with the use of automated external defibrillators in public access defibrillator programmes in comparison with standard resuscitation [16]. The functional state of survival patients in these series are good. The quality of life and the neurological state of the majority of long-term survivals are similar to the general population of the same age, as was observed in a group of 200 out-of-hospital cardiac arrest cases with ventricular fibrillation, with a survival rate to discharge of 42% [17].

In this context, it seems that the statement that resuscitation manoeuvres should always be started in a person who has suffered a sudden cardiac arrest are still applicable [2], unless a DNAR order had been dictated due to the poor recovery possibilities of the patient or that the patient himself/herself or his/her surrogate had given an advanced directive against the move CPR [8].

However, some voices have a different opinion based on the fact that many resuscitation survivors have permanent neurological disability [7] and suggest that resuscitation manoeuvres should not be initiated without a prior informed consent from the patient in which he/she specifically authorises resuscitation in the case of cardiac arrest, to avoid a heavy burden on the family and society in the form of a patient without hope [18]. As is natural, this proposal has been contested because it implies denying the possibility of survival to some patients, mainly favouring those who suffer a cardiac arrest with some particular circumstances which predispose them to a higher chance of success and a low likelihood of neurological impairment [19].

Do Not Attempt Resuscitation Order: Ethical or Legal Issue?

Although it is important to analyse the legal aspects, they can differ from one country to another and may not be clearly defined in their legal regulations, as is the case in Spain and in most European countries [4]. However, the ethical principles are accepted worldwide and they give us a more global guide [4, 9].

The Patient's Autonomy to Decide

Until a few years ago the decision of withholding cardiopulmonary resuscitation was a clinical decision of those in charge of the patient. However, since the Patient Self-Autodetermination Act was promulgated in December 1991, after its approval in the USA Supreme Court in June 25 of 1990, the patients or their surrogates have an important role in taking decisions in the patient's end of life. The Act recognises the right to give priority to the patient's wishes in order to preserve their personal freedom in taking medical decisions. However, the implementation of the patient's autonomy for taking medical decisions has been different from one country to another, due to cultural, religious and sociological reasons [8]. Although the final decisions should obviously be made by the physician in charge, after consulting the patient and the relatives [20], there are, however, numerous factors that influence the patient's decision.

The main factor in taking the decision to accept a DNAR order for the patients is the quality of life after discharge. If it may be restored to the previous level, 90% of the patients wanted resuscitation to be performed, while only a 16% wanted CPR if the possibilities for recovery were poor and only 6% if they would remain in vegetative state [21]. The diagnosis, the age (being older), being more functionally impaired and the patient's anticipation of a worse prognosis are also important factors [22]. The burden of treatment that would be needed to return to current health are also important, but the likelihood of a functional and, even more, a cognitive impairment, are the most important factors that influence the treatment preferences of the seriously ill older persons [23]. Race plays also a role in the patient's decision. In the USA, Hispanics and black patients want to prolong their lives and have a lower rate of DNAR orders than non-Hispanic white patients, regardless of their disease and prognosis [24–25].

Health economics and the way that health care is covered in different countries may also influence a patient's decision to refuse resuscitation. In the USA, treatment decisions are often taken under the influence of insurance coverage rather than the real desires of the patients [26]. Moreover, the cultural context may have an important role in the patient autonomy. In Japan, the family and the physicians' role in ethical decisions at the end of life are greater than that of the patients [27].

Physicians' opinions may differ when faced with the same situation and the physicians' attitudes concerning life support may influence the patient's and relatives' decisions. The medical speciality and the years of experience influence the opinions regarding DNAR orders [28]. Not only the physicians themselves, but the type of hospital where they work influence the patient's decision. In the SUPPORT study, the hospital site was an independent factor associated with patient CPR preferences [22]. The lack of training in communication and in taking decisions at the end of life in the physician's medical education may produce patient insecurity at the moment of taking a decision regarding preferences for CPR [8]. Consensus protocols may assist for taking decisions in life-threatening situations by helping physicians to decide the treatment in these situations [29].

The approach that the decision of a DNAR order should be decided after discussion between the patients and their relatives and the responsible physician to know the patient's desires, is well accepted in USA, however, it is not totally implemented in other countries. In Europe, there is no well established culture of patient autonomy and the proposal to withhold or withdraw life-support measures is usually initiated by the physician in charge. In Spain this rate is as high as 92.9% [30]. This European 'paternalistic approach' by the physicians may indicate that the physician takes the unilateral decision not to perform CPR [31], as well as practice resuscitation manoeuvres in a patient without clear possibilities of a good outcome, without knowing the patient's wishes [32]. This conduct, however, is not uniform in different European countries. In 1999, the written DNAR orders were applied only by 8% of Italian physicians whereas in The Netherlands 91% of the physicians agreed on stating a DNAR order when indicated [33]. Due also to cultural and religious reasons, the physician's decision to perform an unsuccessful CPR may fluctuate from country to country in Europe between 5% and 48% [32].

On some occasions, the physician may even override a DNAR order [20]. This may happen, for instance, in iatrogenic cardiac arrest, especially when it is due to a physician's error [19, 34].

In some situations, the patients are not competent to take decisions or to express their wills. The ICU is one of the contexts where it is harder to determine patients' wishes. Less than 5% of ICU patients have the capacity to take a decision about their end-of-life care [35]. In these cases, relatives or surrogates are the physician's interlocutors to agree a DNAR order. In recent years, in order not to misinterpret the wishes of these patients, advanced directives have been introduced in many countries, such as living wills, and the nomination of selected surrogates, for notifying and discussing about patient end-of-life decisions. However, these have proven to be of little help, mainly because their implementation has been very poor, at least in Europe. In Finland, in a recent study, only 3% of the residents in long-term care facilities have living wills [31]. In one Spanish region, Andalusia, with more than 6 million inhabitants, the Advanced Directive Register had only 252 subjects with living wills registered [36], two years after the Spanish law on patient autonomy and advanced directives had been published [37].

Medical Futility in DNAR

The decision of a DNAR order should be agreed between the patients and/or their relatives or surrogate and the physicians, but sometimes there is disagreement. When the patients or relatives demand full resuscitation and the physicians do not agree, the physicians usually base their opinion on the fact that CPR will be futile [5].

The definition of futility in resuscitation is not clear. In front of one identical theoretical clinical situation the physician's opinions regarding DNAR orders differ among different medical specialities and depend also on the years of experience [28]. Curtis et al. have found evidence of major misunderstandings of the concepts of both quantitative and qualitative futility [38]. Some recommendations have been proposed to help physicians to determine medical futility [29, 39]. In recent years, some voices have claimed a better definition of futility in order to preserve the patient in the case of a unilateral physician decision, taking into account the inconsistency of the futility definition [40]. It has even considered that a unilateral DNAR order taken by an individual physician, without patient or relative agreement, may constitute malpractice and an uncertain legal position [5, 9]. In the USA, the courts have not supported physicians' determinations of futility in these cases [5].

In order to guarantee the best benefit for the patient, an individual physician should never write a DNAR order without an active enquiry into the patient's desires, if they are aware. If they are not aware, the decision should only be taken after a discussion with their relatives or surrogates. In the case of dissent, a neutral process should be initiated in order to resolve the disagreement [41]. Seeking a second opinion may help to clarify the patient's prognosis to the family, or it may require an Ethical Committee consultation to reach a fair decision that would satisfy all [40]. Consensus panel guidelines may assist in taking the decision not to perform CPR [29]. In the recent Statement of the 5th International Consensus Conference in Critical Care on Challenges in end-of-life care in the ICU, whilst recognising that the ultimate responsibility in taking the final decision is in the hands of the physician, recommends a 'shared decision' and an ethical consultation in case of conflict due to disagreement [35].

In some circumstances, futility has been proposed in order to ensure a hypothetical social justice: CPR in the wrong patient may prevent an appropriate treatment in a patient with more possibilities of survival for reasons of lack of resources [4, 42, 43]. However, the physician in his individual decision of proposing a DNAR order should never consider anything other than physiological condition of the patient and the possibilities of an outcome with a good quality of life [44].

Should the Patient's Wishes Always Be Known for Performing CPR?

In most clinical situations of cardiac arrest, the patient's opinion is not known. In out-of-hospital cardiac arrest, the first-responders and the emergency medical services in many of the cases are unaware of the underlying cause of the cardiac arrest. For many years, initiating CPR has been the standard practice in these situations. In a recent review, the main conclusion is that 'after 25 years of do-not-resuscitate orders, it remains reasonable to presume consent and attempt resuscitation for people who have an unexpected cardiopulmonary arrest or for whom resuscitation may have physiologic effect and for whom no information is available at the time as to their wishes' [8].

In others settings, as in hospitals, long-term care facilities, etc., patient's wishes should be more easily come by, as well as the underlying diseases and their prognosis. However, the patients seldom have the opportunity to give their opinion about an end-of-life decision and the physician responsible in most of the cases does not initiate a process to establish a DNAR order either, or indicate the procedures when faced with a cardiac arrest, when it occurs. The rate of written DNAR orders is very different from one country to another, with a wide range, but it is far from optimal even in patients with a high risk of mortality and poor chance of recovery from a cardiac arrest [22, 30, 32, 33]. Here, as well as in out-of-hospital cardiac arrests, guidelines, formal policies, etc, should be stated in order to guarantee the patient benefit, not only in terms of initial survival but also subsequent quality of life [8, 42, 45].

Conclusions

Although autonomy is considered the primary ethical principle in a cardiac arrest situation, it remains difficult to apply. A cardiac arrest is always an emergency situation and the patient's desires are seldom stated beforehand. In this situation, the weight of the ethical principle of beneficence and non-maleficence is the most important [43]. The physicians are obliged in these situations to evaluate the real possibilities of the outcome of resuscitation in a particular patient, actively seek the wishes of the patient, relatives or surrogate, whenever possible. Ideally, the decision should be taken in advance, via a written DNAR order, in agreement with the patient or representatives, always bearing in mind that saving the patient's life is not always the main objective: this remains the restoration of the prior health status [8, 21, 23, 43].

References

1. American Heart Association (1974) Standards and guidelines for cardiopulmonary resuscitation (CPR) and emergency cardiac care (ECC): Medicolegal considerations and recommendations. JAMA 227(Suppl):864–866
2. American Heart Association in collaboration with International Liaison Committee on Resuscitation (2000) Guidelines 2000 for cardiopulmonary resuscitation and emergency cardiovascular care: International consensus on science. Part 2: Ethical aspects of CPR and ECC. Resuscitation 46:17–27
3. Emergency Cardiac Care Committee and Subcommittees, American Heart Association (1992) Guidelines for cardiopulmonary resuscitation and emergency cardiac care. Part VIII: Ethical consideration in resuscitation. JAMA 268:2282–2288
4. Anonymous (1988) Ethical principles in out–of–hospital cardiopulmonary resuscitation. In: Bossaert L (ed) European Resuscitation Council Guidelines for Resuscitation. Elsevier, Amsterdam, pp 206–209
5. Cotler MP (2000) The 'do not resuscitate' order; clinical and ethical rationale and implications. Med Law 19:623–633
6. Eisemberg MS (1990) Cardiac arrest and resuscitation: A tale of 29 cities. Ann Emerg Med 19:179–186
7. Roine RO, Kajaste S, Kaste M (1993) Neurophysiological sequelae of cardiac arrest. JAMA 269:237–242
8. Burns JP, Edwards J, Johnson J et al (2003) Do–not–resuscitate order after 25 years. Crit Care Med 31:1593–1595
9. Snider GL (1991) The do–not–resuscitate order. Ethical and legal imperative or medical decision? Am Rev Respir Dis 143:665–674
10. Eisemberg MS, Mengert T (2001) Cardiac resuscitation. N Engl J Med 344:1304–1313
11. Nichol G, Stiell IG, Laupacis A et al (1999) A cumulative meta–analysis of effectiveness of defibrillator–capable emergency medical services for victims of out–of–hospital cardiac arrest. Ann Emerg Med 34:517–525
12. The Pre–Hospital Arrest Survival Evaluation (PHASE) Study. Lombardi G, Gallagher J, Gennis P (1994) Outcome of out–of–hospital cardiac arrest in New York City. JAMA 271:678–683
13. Peberdy MA, Kaye W, Ornato JP et al (2003) Cardiopulmonary resuscitation of adults in the hospital: a report of 14720 cardiac arrests from the National Registry of Cardiopulmonary Resuscitation. Resuscitation 58:297–308
14. Valenzuela TD, Roe DJ, Nichol G et al (2000) Outcomes of rapid defibrillation by security officers after cardiac arrest in casinos. N Engl J Med 343:1206–1209
15. The PAD Trial Investigators (2003) The public access defibrillation (PAD) trial. Study design and rationale. Resuscitation 56:135–147
16. http://www.nih.gov/news/pr/nov2003/nhlbi–11.htm
17. Bunch TJ, White RD, Gersh BJ et al (2003) Long–term outcomes of out–of–hospital cardiac arrest after successful early defibrillation. N Engl J Med 348:2626–2633
18. Jaffe AS, Landau WM (1993) Death after death: The presumption of informed con-

sent for cardiopulmonary resuscitation – ethical paradox and clinical conundrum. Neurology 43:2173-2178

19. Choudhry NK, Choudhry S, Singer PA (2003) CPR for patients labelled DNR: The role of the limited aggressive therapy order. Ann Intern Med 138:65-68
20. Karnik AM, Brook S (2002) End-of-life issues and do-not-resuscitate order. Who gives the order and what influences the decision? Chest 121:683-686
21. Frankl D, Oye RK, Bellamy PE (1989) Attitudes of hospitalised patients toward life support: a survey of 200 medical inpatients. Am J Med 86:645-648
22. Phillips RS, Wenger NS, Teno J et al (1996) Choices of seriously ill patients about cardiopulmonary resuscitation: correlates and outcomes. Am J Med 100:128-137
23. Fried TR, Bradley EH, Towle VR et al (2002) Understanding the treatment preferences of seriously ill patients. N Engl J Med 346:1061-1066
24. Caralis PV, Davis B, Wright K et al (1993) The influence of ethnicity and race on attitudes toward advanced directives, life-prolonging treatments and euthanasia. J Clin Ethics 4:155-165
25. Shepardson LB, Gordon HS, Ibrahim SA et al (1999) Racial variation in the use of do-not-resuscitate orders. J Gen Intern Med 14:15-20
26. Meier DE, Morrison RS (2002) Autonomy reconsidered. N Engl J Med 346:1087-1089
27. Ruhnke GW, Wilson SR, Akamatsu T et al (2000) Ethical decision making and patient autonomy. A comparison of physicians and patients in Japan and the United Sates. Chest 118:1172-1182
28. Kelly WF, Eliasson AH, Stocker DJ et al (2002) Do specialists differ on do-not-resuscitate decisions? Chest 121:957-963
29. Alexandrov AV, Pullicino PM, Meslin EM et al (1996) Agreement on disease specific criteria for do-not-resuscitate orders in acute stroke. Stroke 27:232-237
30. Esteban A, Gordo F, Solsona JF et al (2001) Withdrawing and withholding life support in the intensive care unit: a Spanish prospective multi-centre study. Intensive Care Med 27:1744-1749
31. Laakkonen ML, Finne-Soveri UH, Noro A et al (2004) Advanced orders to limit therapy in 67 long-term care facilities in Finland. Resuscitation 61:333-339
32. Sprung CL, Cohen SL, Sjokvist P et al (2003) End-of-life practices in European intensive care units. JAMA 290:790-797
33. Vincent JL (1999) Forgoing life support in western European intensive units: The results of an ethical questionnaire. Crit Care Med 27:1626-1633
34. Casarett DJ, Stocking CB, Siegler M (1999) Would physicians override a do-not-resuscitate order when a cardiac arrest is iatrogenic? J Gen Intern Med 14:35-38
35. Carlet J, Thijs LG, Antonelli M et al (2004) Challenges in the end-of-life care in the ICU. Statement of the 5th International Consensus Conference in Critical Care: Brussels, Belgium, April 2003. Intensive Care Med 30:770-784
36. Diario Medico. Viernes, 9 de Julio de 2004, p 10
37. Boletín Oficial del Estado. Ley 41/2002, de 14 de noviembre, básica reguladora de la autonomía del paciente y de derechos y obligaciones en materia de información y documentación clínica. BOE núm.274, 15 de noviembre 2002, pp 40126-40132
38. Curtis JR, Park DR, Krone MR et al (1995) Use of the medical futility rationale in do-not-attempt-resuscitation orders. JAMA 273:124-128
39. Doty WD, Walker RM (2000) Medical futility. Clin Cardiol 23(Suppl. II): II6-II16
40. Anonymous (1995) When is CPR futile? JAMA 273:156-158
41. Biegler P (2003) Should patient consent be required to write a do not resuscitate

order? J Med Ethics 29:359–363

42. Doyal L, Wilsher D (1993) Withholding cardiopulmonary resuscitation: proposals for formal guidelines. BMJ 306:1593–1596
43. Mohr M, Kettler D (1997) Ethical aspects of resuscitation. Br J Anaesth 79:253–259
44. Waisel DB, Truog RD (1995) The cardiopulmonary resuscitation–not–indicated order: futility revised. Ann Intern Med 122:304–308
45. Anonymous (1998) The ethics of resuscitation in clinical practice. A statement on behalf of the European Resuscitation Council, 1994. In: Bossaert L (ed) European Resuscitation Council Guidelines for Resuscitation, Elsevier, Amsterdam, pp 210–217

Molecular Biology in Critical Care: Is It More Than a Look Only?

G. Domínguez-Cherit, J. Gutiérrez, E. Rivero

Basic Concepts in Molecular Genetics

During recent years, molecular genetics have become integrated with all aspects of medicine, and advances in this area may modify clinical daily practice deeply as the basic biological mechanisms of illness are understood. The new concepts have been emerging from the knowledge obtained from the study of the human genome, and thanks to advances in computer technology and molecular engineering and new kind of probes developed.

The basic information has come from learning more about genes and their conformation.

Deoxyribonucleic acid (DNA) encodes all the genetic material for cellular function and replication, and consists of a double-stranded molecule composed of deoxyribose residues and four bases: adenine (A), thymine (T), cytosine (C) and guanine (G). Adenine pairs with thymine and guanine pairs with cytosine. When genetic material is to be used for a cellular process or function, it is transcribed in ribonucleic acid (RNA) which differs by having ribose as sugar and uracile instead of thymine.

By convention, the DNA sequence is read from the 5' to the 3' end of DNA molecule, and the complementary strand is termed anti-sense trend.

There are three form of RNA: messenger RNA (mRNA), transfer RNA (tRNA) and ribosomal RNA (rRNA). Messenger RNA encodes the amino acid sequence to a protein sequence. Amino acids are coded on mRNA by codons consisting of three specific nucleotides, although more than one triplet codon is needed to encode amino acids. Transfer RNA carry specific amino acid to the ribosome to permit translation of the mRNA sequence and form base pairs with mRNA.

Introns are non-coding, intervening DNA sequences that interrupt the sequence of a gene, are subsequently removed to form the final mRNA, and have no known direct role in gene regulation. Polymorphisms within specific introns of genes have been associated with gene expression characteristics and clinical outcome. Promoter sequence occurs at the 5′ end of a given sequence not transcribed to mRNA. These regions serve to regulate tightly the rate of gene transcription binding transcription factors that enhance or repress the rate of transcription.

Restriction endonucleases are bacterial enzymes that recognise specific DNA sequences and cleave to DNA at these specific sites [1].

Polymerase chain reaction is a novel tool to expand genomic material based on three properties: the natural process of double DNA transformation to single strand molecule by heating, the ability of single stranded molecule to form double-strand molecules and the high fidelity of the sequence amplified specific of DNA. This makes it possible to amplify amounts of specific DNAs for experimental or diagnosis purposes.

Genomics describes the entire genome, and analyses the expression pattern of hundreds or thousands of genes. It can be divided into structural genomics, the form that generates and assembles genetic nucleic acid sequences, and functional genomics which evaluates gene function and products using information and reagents from structural genomics with the help of computational analysis and sophisticated statistical methodologies.

Proteomics studies how proteins interact with each other and with other molecules to control complex processes in cells, tissues and organs; it represents the end product of the genome.

Micro array technology is a platform on which are ordered, small arrays of up to thousands of spots which can be used to analyse DNA, proteins or even whole cells. This technology has the potential to provide real time monitoring in critically ill patients. The major drawback is that because of the enormous amount of data collected, even a minuscule error rate may result in unacceptably high levels of false positives.

Genomic technology is now applied to the development of drugs, and understanding drug metabolism, genetic polymorphisms may affect metabolism and thus the efficacy and safety of drug in a given patient.

Gene therapy may include insertion of a normal copy of a gene to replace a defective one, the insertion of an extra copy of a gene to induce protein production or the insertion of a gene to block transcription of messenger RNA.

Some important mechanisms explaining problems such as apoptosis, ischaemia/reperfusion injury and sepsis are becoming daily more understandable, and the knowledge of all the pathophysiology pathways may serve as the first step for treatment, monitoring and course modification [2].

The Evolving Way of Understanding Illness

Traditionally, physicians use the interpretation of symptoms and signs in order to complete a diagnosis of certain diseases, but sometimes their interpretation should be modified according to the evolution over time of each patient.

Nowadays, the knowledge of the most basic mechanism involved in the pathophysiology of the illness may offer the opportunity to have a more accurate diagnosis and a target-directed model of treatment, and using different kinds of markers the efficacy of medicines may be evaluated soon, making it possible to switch quickly to a different therapeutic regimen that perhaps better responds to the specific change in the patient.

Molecular biology has being evolving from just being a basic research model to a more mature practice tool, helping to improve health of patients at the bedside.

We can now make a better approach to the patient, not just through our knowledge of molecular mechanisms but also by monitoring changes suffered in the body.

Some abnormalities in critical care patients nowadays are monitored by very traditional systems; for example, hypoxia determines a reduction in tissue oxygen tension below normal levels, and dysoxia signifies severe hypoxia that can produce cytochrome turnover. Currently, we use insensitive, non-specific indicators such as blood pressure, heart rate, cardiac output, urine output, arterial and mixed venous oxygen saturation, oxygen transport and consumption, hepatic, cardiac and pancreatic enzyme levels and serum lactate levels. In this way, it is usually not possible to determine when hypoxia, ischaemia, dysoxia dysfunctional energy use, frank energy failure or disruption of cellular integrity is occurring in organs or tissue beds [3].

The cellular events involved in the systemic inflammatory response, organ damage and multiple organ failure syndrome are ultimately controlled at the molecular level, while the effects of hypoxia on tissues can be observed at the level of gene expression.

Activation of genes leads to the synthesis of particular sets of proteins and a consequent change in cellular behaviour. These represent potential targets for intervention but they need accurate and early diagnosis. Advances in biotechnology have permitted the identification of specific cytokines and definition of their roles in tissue injury. For example, the association of changes in the expression of p53 gene or p53-associated genes could signal the development of apoptosis before it occurs.

Genetic Polymorphisms

Host response in the presence of illness provides direct evidence of heritable traits, counting with interpersonal differences and allows genetic detection to determine this difference and sometimes form a prognosis based on it.

The innate and acquired immune system is one of the principal players in the response of acute inflammatory states, such as the systemic inflammatory response syndrome (SIRS). SIRS has been defined clinically and is a response to infectious or non-infectious conditions and is frequently followed by a compensatory anti-inflammatory response syndrome (CARS) [4].

Thus we now know that the equilibrium between a pro-inflammatory response and an anti-inflammatory response is responsible for the path followed by the evolution of the patient.

In order to develop new therapies, specific biochemical mediators and cytokines involved in such processes as well as the genetic control mechanism have been targeted. But there have been poor results in human models, including the improper timing of immune altering measures, the complexity of triggering mechanisms, the redundancy of immune activation pathways and the heterogeneity of the patient population being studied.

If a relationship between the genetic constitution of a patient and a response to a major inflammatory stimulus could be established, better injury scoring systems could be devised that predict the clinical trajectory of the patient.

The presence of 'non self' can in part explain microbe-induced SIRS, but in some conditions as ischaemia/reperfusion, pancreatitis, haemorrhagic shock or thermal injury, this model is not sufficient, so it the idea of 'danger signals' has been proposed, such as heat-shock proteins, necrotic cells, capable of inducing the same inflammatory cascade as lipopolysaccharide (LPSs) components of microbes.

The Biological Response

The pro-inflammatory cytokines function in three ways: they induce production of acute phase proteins by the liver, cause an elevation in body temperature and induce vascular permeability and chemo-attraction of other preformed entities in order to induce sequelae such as local inflammation to prevent systemic dissemination.

There are three principle cytokines that mediate the early acute inflammatory response: IL-1, IL-6 and TNF α. IL-1 helps to start the febrile reaction, stimulates early haematopoietic progenitor cells, and triggers prostanoid release. IL-6 causes B cell proliferation and hepatic synthesis of induced acute proteins. TNF α induces a procoagulant state, stimulates neutrophil recruitment and activation and also in conjunction with IL-1 stimulates anti-inflammatory cytokines IL-10, IL-12, and IL-18.

Links between genetics and host response, and between genetic markers and systemic diseases have been established. While much of the genome is conserved in all members of the species, 1% is repeatedly and reproducibly variable at frequencies higher than random mutations; these areas are called polymorphism. Strictly, these variances are stable in the genome. Common examples are single nucleotide polymorphism (SNPs) and variable number of tandem repeats (VNTRs).

Some of the most studied polymorphism corresponds to the gene cluster that encodes for TNFα and TNFβ on chromosome 6 within the HLA class – III locus. TNFα is produced by macrophages and TNFβ predominantly by lymphocytes. The TNFα gene is highly conserved and has few polymorphisms; one of them, at position – 308, is a guanine (G) in 80% of people, and 20% population have instead adenine (A), the sequence with G is known as TNF1 and the A is TNF 2 allele. Since each person has two copies of the gene, the relative frequencies of G/G, G/A, and A/A are 65-80%, 15-25%, and 2-5%. TNF2 allele has been associated with an increase in TNFα production and some studies found a correlation of mortality higher in patients with at least a copy of TNF2 allele (71.4 vs. 42.6%) in patients with septic shock. In patients with septic shock, Feezor et al. found mortality for homozygous for TNFB2 allele of 81% opposed to heterozygous who had 42% [5].

Interleukin 1 encodes for 3 proteins IL-1αβ IL-1 and IL-1ra which provide the platform for the activation of MyD88 and IRAK, whose phosphorylation leads to translocation of nuclear factor kB. IL-1ra seems to offer some protection in patients with sepsis but on the other hand the risk of developing immune-mediated diseases is higher in patients with IL-1 ra A2 allele. IL-6 has both pro and anti-inflammatory effects; high levels of it had been considered as adversely affecting allograft solid organ transplantation recipients. The ethnicity study showed that 98% of African-Americans are high IL-6 producers while only 84% Caucasians were similarly classified. Nuclear factor kB (NF-kB) is a DNA binding protein that incites high-level transcription of pro-inflammatory genes. Its monocyte production has been associated to end organ failure and predicted survival for septic patients. Toll-like receptor 4 (TLR4) is the major receptor for LPS and gram negative bacteria; one known mutation at position 299 may predispose the bearer to septic shock.

The Danger Model, Distress, Damage Destruction, and Death

The original concept of immune system recognition just between self and non-self products should be reanalysed in order to obtain a better explanation of the protective model. The danger model has now established the fact that the immune system is more concerned with danger and potential destruction than the distinction between self and non self. Basically, the new concept supports the idea that distressed cells send alarm signals that activate its local antigen presenting cells (APCs), and on the other hand 'pattern recognition receptors' (PRRs) are receptors on APCs that may activate them by recognising bacterial products such as (LPS), and other different organisms based on a non-self evolutionary discriminate code. These signals sustain the activation of helper cells and B cells in order to prevent its death. The nature of these danger signals still need to be determined because it has not been possible to recognise them fully, but generally each protein that apoptotic cells maintain inside and in necrotic cells get outside free may serve as signal.

In case of critical care patients the treatments against pro or anti-inflammatory stages in sepsis patients have failed, basically because the answer should be in the difficult to characterise the underlying defect, this is understood as the immune status of each patient.

Some methods proposed to define the immune status are:

- Cellular stimulation: immunoparalysis is the condition subsequent to down regulation of TNF, IL-1, IL-6 and IL-8 expression in patients with septic shock; the identification of this condition by monitoring the degree of HLA DR expression may help following response to treatment.
- Circulating cytokines: some cytokines have been proposed as markers in sepsis response – maybe the most consistently reported cytokine with prognosis is IL-6. However, it is not exclusively of sepsis.
- Other markers: C reactive protein and the peptide procalcitonin, elastase and neopterin are molecules now studied in order to evaluate response of treatment in sepsis patients and discriminate between infective or not stage.

The future of the treatment is based on the capability to distinguish the immune status and based on this start a pro inflammatory or anti inflammatory strategy [6].

Apoptosis and Critical Illness

The great problem after activating the process to protect the organism against an external challenge is the return to a state of quiescence in order to restore normal homeostasis. Impossibility to return to this state may be the cause of more injury; quite recently, attention has been focused on this process of resolution determined by the programmed cell death: apoptosis.

Apoptosis is a physiological process that results from adequate embryogenesis, and it regulates gut and skin epithelial cell turnover, andis critical to normal immunity to remove inflammatory cells such as neutrophils and selective deletion of T cells directed against self antigens. The abnormal process of these phenomena may lead to autoimmunity diseases, neurodegenerative diseases and pathogenesis of acquired immunodeficiency syndrome.

Necrosis and apoptosis are quite different but both result in cell death. In apoptosis, we are in the presence of an active process that requires energy and where nuclear chromatin is condensed and nuclear fragmentation in membrane bound apoptotic bodies take place, cytostructural and reparative proteins are degraded, the cell membrane remains intact and some phosphatidyl serines residues are expressed on cell surface to mark it for phagocytosis by macrophages. Biochemical changes were first studied in the soil nematode C. elegans identified as the first homolog in humans for bcl-2 protein-, which has been identified as part of a family capable of promoting or inhibiting apoptosis. Some cysteine proteases with cleavage target in an Asp-X residue are known now as caspases, and are divided into three families of inactive precursors of apoptosis that may be activated by autocatalytic cleavage. The activation of caspase cascade can be made by different pathways, one of them implicating modifications in mitochondrial transmembrane potential, which may lead to uncoupling of the respiratory chain with reduced ATP production, and also the contact of cytochrome c with apoptosis protease activating factor–1, which recruits and activate caspase 9, initiating a caspase cascade [7].

Another way of activating caspases includes type 1 membrane protein receptors including Fas, tumor necrosis factor receptor p55, CD40, DR3/TRAMP and related apoptosis inducing ligand (TRAIL), which activates membrane associated proteins known as death-inducing signalling complex (DISC) which activates caspase 8 and initiates the cascade. Altered apoptosis may induce liver failure, tubular necrosis, or gastrointestinal alterations. In critical patients, it may induce T cell anergy in contrast to polymorphonuclear delayed apoptosis.

Ischaemia/Reperfusion Injury

Many mechanism are implicated in ischaemia/reperfusion injury (I/R): first the depletion of energy intracellular conditions, a poor ionic pumping function with ingress of calcium and sodium ions into ischaemic cells. Inflammatory changes take place in endothelium going I/R. Reactive oxygen species (ROS) such as superoxide, hydrogen peroxide and hydroxyl radical are produced as well as overwhelming scavenging systems as superoxide dismutase (SOD), glutathione peroxidase and catalase.

ROS can be produced by different intracellular mechanisms such as mitochondrial transport chains or as a product of cyclooxygenase and lypoxygenase pathways. By xanthine oxidase or NAD(P)H oxidase, and by reaction of hydrogen peroxidase and iron or copper atoms to produce hydroxyl radicals. Superoxide can be metabolised to hydrogen peroxide by SOD.

Transgenic mice overexpressing SOD had demonstrated a reduction in I/R injury.

The relationship between apoptosis and I/R injury is very close, and some studies are directed to the administration of caspase inhibitors in order to reduce ischaemia injuries, as in the case of neurological resuscitation.

In addition to previous mediators, this complement system also constitutes an important cause of I/R injury. The complement is composed of more than 30 proteins that circulates as inactive zymogens, proteolytic activation in a cascade finish in the membrane attack complex consisting of the components C5, C6, C7, C8 and polymeric C9 which can induce cell lysis. Immune complex containing IgM or IgG are activators of classical pathway, also activated by bacterial components, and C reactive protein. Two other ways can induce complement the mannan binding lecithin and the alternative pathway. All three ways finish activating C3. The most toxic complement activation products are generated at the level of C5, and studies inhibiting this protein by monoclonal antibodies diminish reperfusion injury [8].

Recent trends of therapeutic possibilities have focused on the function of the mitochondrial inner membrane which is disrupted, and mitochondrial uncoupled in case of the opening of mitochondrial permeability transition pore (MPTP). This options include Cyclosporine A that inhibits MPTP in isolated heart preparation- the protection declines at concentrations higher than $0.2\mu M$. Other options include low pH maintaining an acidic extracellular pH during reoxigenation after a period of anoxia, which may protect cells from damage. By contrast, acid pH during ischaemic phase is detrimental because it enhances Na^+/H^+ exchanges with greater loading of the heart with Na^+ and Ca^+.

Two other drugs studied in case of reperfusion injury are: Pyruvate and Propofol.

The protective effects of Pyruvate may in part result from its capacity as a free radical scavenger, but it also is a good respiratory substrate that does not depend on ATP dependent phosphorylation prior to metabolism, and may produce a high mitochondrial membrane potential and increased mitochondrial $NADH/NAD^+$ and $NADPH/NADP^+$ ratios.

Propofol is an anaesthetic agent that can act as a free radical scavenger and inhibits MPTP, the mechanism includes inhibition of plasma membrane calcium channels [9].

Coagulation System and Inflammatory Mediators

Thrombin generation in systemic circulation promotes inflammatory responses by inducing platelet aggregation through microcirculation activate P selectin that induces cell rolling and attachment of white cells to capillaries that contribute to further vascular damage. The levels of antithrombin III, protein C and protein S are reduced in severe sepsis and cause an adverse outcome. Therapy with recombinant protein C has proved of benefit for regulating coagulation cascade and reducing pro-inflammatory signals with increased survival of septic patients.

Cell Adhesion Molecules and Inflammation

Interaction between leukocytes and endothelial cells is regulated by expression of cell adhesion molecules (CAM). These molecules mediate the attachment between cells and the extracellular matrix.

CAM also produces functional responses by their interaction to intracellular domains. Therapies regulating CAM expression may be of benefit in order to diminish neuthrophil migration and local damage for release of inflammatory mediators Moreover, CAM molecules also assist the reparative process controlling differentiation of epithelial, stromal and vascular cells.

There are some adhesion family molecules involved in rolling, adhesion and transmigration of leukocytes.

Selectins: E selectin, P selectin and L selectin are glycoproteins bound to an epithelial growth factor domain, and small cytoplasmic domain. Neuthrophils, monocytes and lymphocytes bind all three selectins.

Integrins, intracellular adhesion molecules and cadherins are adhesion molecules involved in signalling leukocytes migration.

The blocking of this mechanism may offer a reduction in mortality in end toxaemic models. Some interventions such as using corticosteroids, anti cytokine agents, and nitric oxide inhibit adhesion molecules.

Trials in rheumatoid arthritis, inflammatory bowel disease and multiple sclerosis are promising, although sepsis trials are very poor [10].

Gender and Immunity

Gender has shown differences in immune response following haemorrhagic shock. In laboratory preparations, female mice tend to support haemorrhagic shock differently to males, with less gut dysfunction and lung injury.

Increased thymic apoptosis is also related with gender but these differences are lost with age as females loose their sex steroid levels.

Female sex steroids have stimulatory effects on cell mediated immunity, and 17 β estradiol can stimulate macrophage function and T cell activity. Dehydroepiandrosterone (DHEA) has estrogenic effects on male mice and prevents the splenic suppression of immune function.

Prolactin restores suppression of T cell responses in male mice following haemorrhage shock, and decreased mortality after bacterial insult; a single dose of metoclopramide may improve cell-mediated immune response [11]. The only exception appears to be after burn injuries where oestrogen is immunosuppressive. These observations may open a variety of possibilities for treatment with hormones or specific blockade of dopamine agonist.

References

1. Shanley T, Wong H (2003) Molecular genetics in pediatric intensive care unit. Crit Care Clin 3:577–594
2. Kohli–Seth R, Oropello JM (2000) The future of bedside monitoring. Crit Care Clin 16(4):557578, vii–viii
3. Hopf HW (2003) Molecular diagnostics of injury and repair responses in critical illness: what is the future of 'monitoring' in the intensive care unit? Crit Care Med 31(8 Suppl):S518–S523
4. Bone RC, Grodzin CJ, Balk RA (1997) Sepsis: a new hypothesis for pathogenesis of the disease process. Chest 112:235–243
5. Feezor R, Moldawer L (2003) Genetic polymorphisms, functional genomics and the host inflammatory response to injury and inflammation. In: Cynober L, Moore F (eds) Nutrition and critical care, Karger AG, Basel, pp 15–37
6. Vincent JL (2002) The immune response in critical illness: excessive, inadequate or dysregulated. In Marshall J, Cohen J (eds) Immune response in the critically ill, Springer, Berlin Heidelberg, pp 12–21
7. Taneja R, Yue L, Marshall C (2002) Programmed cell death (apoptosis) and the immunologic derrangements of critical illness. In: Marshall J, Cohen J (eds) Immune response in the critically ill, Springer, Berlin, Heidelberg, pp 264–279
8. Ciurana C, Hack C (2002) Molecular mechanisms of complement activation during ischemia and reperfusion. In: Vincent JL (ed) Intensive Care Medicine annual update 2002. Springer, Berlin, Heidelberg, pp 39–49
9. Halestrap A. Toole O, Lim K (2002) The mitochondrial permeability transition: a 'pore' way to die. In: Evans T, Fink M, Vincent JL (eds) Mechanism of organ dysfunction in critical illness, Springer, Berlin, Heidelberg, pp 1739
10. Finney S, Evans T, Burke-Gaffney A (2002) Cell adhesion molecules and leukocyte trafficking in sepsis. In: Vincent JL (ed) Intensive Care Medicine annual update 2002. Springer, Berlin,Heidelberg, pp 23–38
11. Schwacha M, Samy A, Chaudry I (2002) Gender and cell mediated immunity following trauma, shock and sepsis. In: Vincent JL (ed) Intensive Care Medicine annual update 2002, Springer, Berlin, Heidelberg, pp 50–61

Resource Management and Audits in Intensive Care Medicine

A.O. GALLESIO

The concept of management is often reduced to accountable administrative processes. This misconception leads to considering that the main goal of an intensive care unit director is to control the magnitude and the final results of intensive care unit (ICU) costs. This is a serious error because it leaves aside the fact that all the steps in the administrative process – purchasing supplies, payments of wages, financial programme, accounting entries, charging of delivered service, costs and balance – are a mirror in terms of monetary units of the resource-consuming process that is necessary for the life support and care of the critically ill patient; the whole administrative process will always be subordinated to medical and nursing interventions.

To achieve its mission, the multidisciplinary task group operating in an ICU use advanced technology, equipment and drugs that are manipulated in a coherent way: mechanical ventilation, analgesia and a sedation process is an example of a highly-integrated assistance process; the results of every process should ideally be capable of being assessed through objective indicators. *Therefore, we call resources to the multidisciplinary human group working in the ICU and to the technology, supplies and medicines, that are necessary to carry out the support of the critical ill patient.*

The administrative instances must adequately mirror the assistance process and provide everything that is necessary for achieving good results. This includes buying and delivering technology and supplies, getting adequate financial support, paying wages and fees, recording movements in accounting books, calculating balances and costs, and drawing up the future budget for renewing resources in order to assure process continuity. *The main role of the ICU director is the management of all these resources.* It is important to remark that the main stress in management must be focused on the development, training and satisfaction of the ICU personnel, since they are in last instance responsible for using resources in order to accomplish their task effectively. *We may thus define management in its broad meaning as the set of activities implemented by the directive board of the unit in order to get a suitable use of resources within a comprehensible organisation that achieves the best results for the established goals of life support for the critically ill patient.*

After evidencing the difference between the management and administrative process, it is now necessary to define some concepts which, coming from the economy, are useful as a basic knowledge for the development of a suitable management and resource utilisation control task. These concepts are: value, costs, prices and market.

Costs

We understand costs as the quantification in monetary units of resource consumption during the assistance and caring delivery process. Applying this concept to the scope of intensive care units, it includes payment of employees' wages and professional fees, supplies, pharmaceuticals, medicinal gases, preventive maintenance, repairing and amortisation of buildings and equipment, general hospital expenses, indirect costs of the institution (light, electricity, central administration, etc).

Prices

By the term 'price', we intend a given amount of monetary units paid by the customer to obtain a service. Although the prices of a service in the public or private sector tend in long term periods to reflect the costs of the services, this is not always true; prices are usually influenced by some other variables. The conditions in which a service should be fulfilled and the price itself are agreed generally through a contract that has legal force. The main factors that determine the price are summarised below:

- Structure of costs
- Supply and demand forces in the market
- State regulations: this item is particularly important in the health area, since health is considered one of the inherent rights of the human being and its value is so high that its price cannot be tied only to market supply and demand laws and influences
- General economic factors, mainly variation in the national currency value, and global and national economic crises

Value and prices are different concepts but they are often confused. *We understand value as the subjective desire that the society gives to the acquisition of a good or service and the quality with which it is delivered to the customer.* This concept does not fit into a purely economic definition because it includes a human need. The greater the subjective importance that each individual gives to obtaining a service, the greater will be the value of that service. Obviously, health is a value desired by every human being, and therefore its social price will be always very high. The importance that the whole of society gives to different services will determine its social value. It is easy to appreciate that health, along with education, are two of the most demanded social values in all human societies throughout history.

The customer may perceive the service differently, and it may happen that the quality of the delivered service be perceived as the minimum expected or it may reach the average expectations that the population has for a similar one. But it may also happen that the service delivery surpasses expectations; if this is so, the user receives more than he had expected, and it is said that this particular service has generated value; indeed, it is so, because value has a subjective component. If patients remain very satisfied with the perceived quality of a service, it is customary they comment on their experience, and the experience of many users expands the knowledge that the population as a whole has of certain services. This leads to a better positioning vis-à-vis the public and private health financial agents or – which amounts to the same thing – a better position in the market. All attempts to develop a continuous quality improvement programme to offer a better service will add value to the ICU. We have already seen that the components that comprise the price conformation often have nothing to do with cost structure; in fact, a reasonable handling of costs and the quality of the services offered to the users promotes the institution among the population that potentially will use these services: an increase in the social preference of a certain institution or service increases its value and in the long term this preference will influence the prices. So a correct resource and quality management of services delivered in the ICU are two inseparable parts of a common process for achieving our mission.

To complete these general concepts, it is necessary now to talk about the market concept and the particularities it has in the health area. *Market is the space where goods and services compete for the preference of clients and users. On the basis of the relationship of the amount of supply and demand services and the state regulations, a price is established in the market.* We have already seen that frequently the health market is strongly regulated by the state. Besides this regulation, the health market has also some peculiarities that deserve a further analysis. In any area of human activity, a customer who wishes to acquire a service informs himself of the possibilities existing in the market from relatives, friends or other people who have acquired a similar service and then usually takes a personal decision. Also, in most cases, the user is the one who pays for the delivered service. Some services offered by the state, especially education and health, offer fewer possibilities of a personal selection. In these cases, service improvement must be claimed through political, legal or social actions.

Furthermore, even in the private area the health market is not typical:

- Frequently, the service user may not be able to choose, or he may do so only in a limited way, particularly in the ICU where critical patients are transferred following a medical decision. Generally, a patient who is in an urgent situation is not able to choose where to be transferred. Furthermore, the selection has been made previously by the third-party payer through a contract of which the user is usually unaware.
- Secondly, those who sign a contract with a medical services provider and pay for the offered service are not the patients, but a third-party payer. It is the state through public budgets that pays for medical attendance of its citizens in public hospitals. The terms of these contracts and the services that must be delivered free-of-charge to the customer are in most cases not completely known by patients. This event is almost dramatically out-standing in the intensive care area: the patient and his family will rely immediately on an unknown service that has to deal with the mission of preserving the life of a beloved person. Conflicts may originate if the ICU staff are not trained in dealing with these difficult challenges. Usually, patients and their families demand that everything must be done for their relatives admitted to the unit. This is a rational claim in the majority of cases, but when we are faced with an unrecoverable life-threatening episode, an unjustified use of resources may follow, and this must be resolved only through an adequate and compassionate persuasion.
- Third, those who determine the total charge of the service are not the patients or the third-party payer, but the ICU team responsible for the patient care. Costs and use of resources are mainly bound to the case mix risk admitted and to the length of stay in the ICU, but on the basis of an average cost assessed according to this case mix, it will be the intervening health team that, in agreement with an institutional assistance culture, will determine the level of resources used and therefore the costs.

Human Resources

A resources utilisation analysis is necessary for auditing its rational use. Services in general and particularly medicine are characterised by intensive requirements for human resources, and this is in opposition to what has been happening in the manufacturing industry, where the introduction of micro-processor technology and installation of entire robotic production lines has replaced human work to a great extent. Medical diagnostic and therapeutic intervention and nursing care cannot be replaced by machines. A nurse/patient relationship of 1:2 has been advised as necessary for an ICU and specialised medical staffing with a 24 hour permanence in the ICU has also been shown to result in better outcomes and decreased costs [1]. When transforming hours of human resource workforce into wages paid, a proportion near 35-50% of the total cost is reached.

The health team involved in the operative management of an ICU and the attendance of critical ill patients has been multidisciplinary since the first specialised ICU emerged. Intensive care is one of the areas, in medicine, where medical, nursing, technician, engineering and administrative personnel become more interdependent; each professional area has its own function and responsibility profile, clearly differentiating the one from the other, but necessary for a co-ordinated team operation. Usually the ICU health team is made up of specialised nurses and physicians, but technicians also have an important role in carrying out mechanical ventilation and homodynamic interventions. Specialised nutritionists, pharmacists, physiotherapists and others specialities complete the necessary team for achieving the goal of recovering the critically ill patient. Perhaps the most important role in the ICU is fulfilled by the nursing team; the interaction of the medical staff with the nursing team is perhaps one of the most important aspects of ICU management. The Intensive Care Units must be headed by a specialist in Intensive Care and the head of the nursing team head should also have training in intensive care nursing. We will now analyse some aspects of the responsibilities of the personnel assigned to the ICU.

Medical Team

Medical responsibilities in the ICU are essentially to provide life support for the critically ill patient through diagnostic and therapeutic interventions that allow him to recover from organ and system insufficiencies. The daily follow-up of patients admitted to the unit is the responsibility of the medical staff who must also watch over the orders to be fulfilled correctly. The ICU director has the responsibility of co-ordinating the whole medical process and the global assistance and administrative management.

- ICU Director: This responsibility requires a medical professional, specialising in intensive care medicine. The leading medical and administrative responsibility of the ICU must ideally not be shared with other staff levels except with the chief of nurses. It is inferred from the management definition that this is a non-delegable responsibility of the ICU director as he is the individual who must answer for the quality of services that are delivered to patients.
- Staff Physicians: the ICU director must be supported by physicians qualified in intensive care. Their number must be determined on the base of

the number of ICU beds and complexity of the ICU. An assistant doctor for each 6 to 8 beds is to be recommended according to the type of ICU: the numbers may differ according to whether a coronary, surgical, medical or specialised unit.

-   Physician on duty 24 hours: the presence of a 24 hour physician on duty in the ICU will depend on hospital organisation. Large university affiliated hospitals with many residents in training and fellows, and specialised well-trained nurses and technicians are capable of running without an intensive care doctor remaining continuously in the unit; however, a specialist in intensive care must be on call in the institution or nearby. This is not the case in developing or undeveloped countries where well-trained nurses are extremely scarce and where respiratory and homodynamic technicians on duty in the ICU do not exist at all. Intensive care specialised physicians should remain in the unit in these cases.
-   Training physician: Ideally doctors in training must have responsibilities limited to their experience and to the ability level they have reached. They must be supervised by a permanent ICU staff physician. It is useful to stress here that frequent departures from this concept are often seen in large institutions dedicated to continuous medical education with extensive residence and fellow programmes. Many times, trainees are left with excessive responsibilities for patient management that do not accord with their training level.

Nursing Team

The role of nurses in the ICU are complementary with and of the same importance as medical tasks. Its aims are different and referred to the diagnostic of patient care needs and also to the interventions necessaries to carry out that care. This task is different to medical responsibilities which are mainly the diagnosis and therapeutic intervention necessary to preserve life and to maintain an adequate medical – patient – family relationship. The number and skills of nursing personnel in an ICU is summarised below:

-   Chief of nurses: The nurse staff should be handled by a nurse with certified qualifying training in Intensive Care. As the director of the unit, he or she should have the responsibility for planning, organising, controlling, implementing and carrying out the audit of the quality of care delivered to the patients.
-   Nurses: They should ideally be certified specialised nurses trained for intensive care. The number of nurses should be adapted to the number of ICU beds and to the patient case mix risk admitted to the area. A relation of one nurse to each two patients has been recommended by many authors. Nevertheless, this concept has been criticised for its inflexibility.

The number of beds handled by one nurse must be calculated according to the levels of care delivered to the patient.

The European Society of Intensive Care Medicine classifies nursing care into three levels as may be seen in Table 1. The most commonly used score to establish the magnitude of the task to be carry out by the nurse team comes from the Simplified Therapeutic Intervention Scoring System [2] (TISS) that originally proposed 76 items based on complexity of care to calculate the score for each patient; this method has been the most used worldwide to determine patient needs and amount of nursing care. This list was reduced to 28 items (TISS28) by Miranda et al. [3-4]. The items used in this new simplified score and the values assigned to each intervention may be seen in Table 2; it was stressed that one nurse cannot carry out more than 40-50 TISS points. Our own experience shows us that this statement is true. We have also further categorised patients in our ICU through a risk scale:

A. Monitoring: Low-risk patients that only require monitoring that cannot be carried out in other hospital areas.
B. High risk: Patients that currently do not need life support, but do have a high risk of requiring it in the next few hours, either because of their basic illness or of a severe chronic comorbidity: (COPD, cardiac insufficiency, etc.)
C. Critically ill: patient requiring at least one vital organ support.
D. Prolonged critically ill: Patient requiring at least one vital organ function support for more than 72 hours.

Combining this scale with TISS 28 and taking into account some special situations, we have calculated on a twice-daily basis the needs of nursing care for the whole unit according to the following schedule:

– TISS > 46: One nurse per bed
– TISS 18-46: One nurse per two beds, except patients isolated for epidemiological reasons or postoperative transplanted patients with mechanical ventilation
– TISS < 18: In a patient staying in the ICU only for monitoring: one nurse per four beds

Table 1. Bed Nurse Relation Care Levels

Care Level	Nurse/patient relationship
III (Highest)	1/1
II	1/1.6
I (Lowest)	1/3

Recently Miranda et al. [5] reassessed the TISS 28 score. They support a different concept as they maintain that time spent in many nursing activities is not necessarily related to the complexity of care. TISS 28 was mainly based on the type of intervention and not on the actual time that is necessary to carry out a particular care intervention. Many nursing activities are not necessarily related to severity of illness, and cost-effectiveness studies require an accurate evaluation of nursing activities. Five new items and 14 sub-items describing nursing activities in the intensive care unit were added to the list of therapeutic interventions. New activities accounted for 60% of the average nursing time; the new scoring system, Nursing Activities Score (NAE), explained 81% of the work nursing time vs. 43% in the TISS 28. It is necessary to validate this new score in a new sample and in different populations.

Table 2. Simplified Therapeutic Intervention Scoring System

Interventions	Points
Standard monitoring	
Hourly vital signs, regular registration and calculation of fluid balance	5
Laboratory. Biochemical and microbiological investigations	1
Single medication, any route (IV, PO, IM, etc.)	2
Multiple intravenous medications (more than 1 drug, single shots, or continuously)	3
Routine dressing changes. Care and prevention of decubitus and daily dressing change	1
Frequent dressing changes (at least one time per each nursing shift) and/or extensive wound care	1
Care of drains. All (except gastric tube)	3
Cardiovascular Support	
Single vasoactive medication. Any vasoactive drug	3
Multiple vasoactive medications. More than1 vasoactive drug, disregard type and dose.	4
Intravenous replacement of large fluid losses. Fluid replacement > 3 litres per square metre per day, disregard type of fluid administered	4
Peripheral arterial catheter	5
Left atrium monitoring. Pulmonary artery flotation catheter with or without cardiac output measurement	8
Central venous line	2
Cardiopulmonary resuscitation after arrest in the past 24 hours (single precordial percussion not included)	3
Specific Interventions	
Single specific interventions in the ICU. Naso or orotracheal intubation, introduction of a pacemaker, cardioversion, endoscopies, emergency surgery	

in the past 24 hours, gastric lavage. Routine interventions without consequences to the clinical condition of the patient, such as radiographs, echography, ECG, dressings or introduction of venous or arterial catheters, are not included   3

Multiple specific interventions in the ICU. More than one, as described above   5

Specific interventions outside of ICU. Surgery or diagnostic procedures   5

Ventilatory Support
Mechanical ventilation. Any form of mechanical or assisted ventilation with or without PEEP; with or without muscle relaxants; spontaneous breathing with PEEP)   5

Supplementary ventilatory support. Breathing spontaneously through endotracheal tube without PEEP; supplementary oxygen by any method except if mechanical ventilation parameters apply   2

Care of artificial airways. Endotracheal tube or tracheostoma   1

Treatment for improving lung function. Thorax physiotherapy, incentive spirometry, inhalation therapy, intratracheal suctioning   1

Renal Support
Haemofiltration techniques. Dialytic techniques   3

Quantitative urine output measurement   2

Active diuresis (e.g. furosemid > 0.5 mg/kg/day for overload)   3

Neurological Support
Measurement of intracranial pressure   4

Metabolic Support
Treatment of complicated metabolic acidosis/alkalosis   4

Intravenous hyperalimentation   3

Enteral feeding. Through gastric tube or other GI route (e.g. jejunostomy)   2

TISS-28 =
TISS-28 = SUM (points for activities performed)

Time of nurse's care =
(One TISS-28 point equals 10.6 minutes of each 8 h nurse's shift)

TISS-76 correlation =
(Correlation between TISS-28 and TISS-76: r = 0.93, r2 = 0.86)
(TISS-28) = 3.33 + 0.97* (TISS-76)

Pharmaceuticals

Medication is an important component of ICU resource utilisation. The national costs of pharmaceuticals in the US has been calculated as rising from 6% to 15% yearly [6] since 1997; more than 70% of this increase in costs is due to new drugs approval [7]. Pharmaceuticals represent 4 to 7% of hospital expenses [8]. The impact of this increase is even more important in the ICU, as drug utilisation in these areas reaches 38.4% of total pharmaceutical hospital costs and is currently increasing faster than hospital drugs costs: 12% vs. 6% [6]. The cost of ICU drug therapies should not be viewed only in terms of acquisition costs; adverse drug effects (ADEs) in the ICU have also a significant impact on hospital costs. Although the rate of preventable and potential ADEs are greater in ICU than non ICU patients, the event rates are no different when adjusted for the number of drugs administrated. These results suggest that methods that reduce the overall number of drugs used in the ICU are a way to reduce the incidence of ADEs.

The pharmaceuticals component in ICU costs, measured as a percentage of total costs, is different depending on ICU complexity. It also varies in different areas of the world. A country's health system organisation and general economic conditions greatly influence pharmaceutical costs. ICU pharmacy charges account for 11 to 35% of total ICU charges. This percentage may vary with the impact of other components in the ICU costs scheme; in particular, staff wages and medical fees have an important impact in ICU costs because human resources are intensively used in this context. Wages and fees vary greatly between countries and also between world and national regions, so, the higher these components are, the more the pharmaceutical percentage weight will decrease in the total costs; inversely if salaries and fees are low, the impact of drugs will be relatively higher. In our country, pharmaceuticals account for approximately 35% of total ICU costs, while employee wages represent approximately another 34%.

The bulk of drugs used in the ICU are associated with only a few therapeutic procedures. Approximately 80% of the total drug utilisation is related to blood volume expansion, blood component transfusion, analgesia and sedation, antibiotics, gastric H^+ secretion inhibitors and heparin. All of these therapeutic interventions have precise aims that can be seen in Table 3.

Table 3. Drug utilisation

Drugs	Therapeutic intervention
Colloid and crystalloids	Blood volume expansion
Blood components	Transfusions
Analgesics and sedatives	Pain management Sedation for adapting to mechanical ventilation
Gastric H+ secretion inhibitors	Prevention and treatment of gastrointestinal bleeding
Heparins	Prevention of deep venous thrombosis and pulmonary thromboembolism

The main way to control and audit use of pharmaceuticals is to establish precise prescription protocols together with setting up an educational programme. These actions must be completed with an information-gathering-programme and an internal ICU or institutional audit system in order to assess the performance of protocol fulfilment.

Audits of resource utilisation in terms of drugs, general supplies and technology, needs for rationale guides and protocols that should be followed by the ICU team involved in the critical ill patient care process and, additionally, a continuous quality-improvement programme will help set up an adequate control of resources.

Traditional styles of practising medicine are being questioned on a worldwide level. Criticism is being levelled from a social, bioethical and economic point of view, focussing on the sharp increases in medical costs. Access to services is frankly unequal, violating basic principles of distributive equity. Questions such as: 'why costs don't increase in line with an improvement in results' or 'why costs vary so much between different institutions, regions and countries' still have no straight answers. New contractual modalities have impelled those who provide medical services to question themselves about this broad variability in attention patterns based on individual experience. A consequence has been the development of documents to describe standards of cares supported by evidence-based medicine; the intention is to decrease variability in medical behaviour. Four main types of documents have been developed: a) Standards of practice; b) Orientative flow charts; c) Guidelines and d) Protocols.

Standards of Practice (SP): They must be seen as rules that define an acceptable minimum standard of a practice the violation of which is generally associated with a bad praxis. An example of standard of practice is the use of sterile techniques in invasive interventions. Standards of practice are formulated as general rules that allow a great variability in protocols design, so that the standard be easily satisfied.

Flow charts: These show the path of successive actions, designed on the basis of logical flow charts, and integrate several aspects of the patient attendance process in a coherent plan that allows a linear continuity. Generally, they include several departments and are specific for a certain pathology. Examples of flow charts are the management of trauma and stroke patients. They tend to be general and they retain a great flexibility in order to be usable for many different situations.

Clinical guides (Guidelines): They are designed to be general enough to be flexible; they consist of a series of recommendations. These recommendations are explicit, but often they use general terms of the type: to consider some kind of diagnostic or therapeutic intervention; they are usually specific to diseases and situations. Examples of guidelines are those written for the diagnosis and treatment of acquired community pneumonia, unstable angina, etc. If they were too specific they could not include the diversity of scenarios that they try to summarise.

Protocols: These are much more specific. They are explicit in instructions and can be followed by medical nurses and other professionals. An example of an ICU protocol is mechanical ventilation in the SDRA. They are specific for a population of patients and for a certain hospital or institution. As an example, a weaning protocol may work well in a multipurpose UCI and not so well in a cardiovascular recovery room. Many protocols refer to drugs frequently used in the ICU: prevention of gastrointestinal bleeding and DVT, analgesia and sedation are all examples of protocols used for controlling the utilisation of drugs in the units. The protocols must have a high level of consensus because they limit the independence of the physician and nurses to decide by themselves. A careful plan of human resources education is always necessary for their implementation. Frequently, since they are specific to procedures, they can form part of several flow charts.

Technology

Technology is an integral part of the ICU structure and must be based on unit complexity and case mix risk admitted to the unit. Definition of the technology to be incorporated is a responsibility of the ICU director but its definition should be discussed by an institutional committee helping him with the technical aspects and opportunities offered in the market. Only few hospitals have written policies for incorporating technology. Written policies must take into account the institution's vision, mission and strategic plan.

Frequently, technology incorporation results in a struggle between the ICU director who defines which technology is necessary and the administrative area that tries to discourage its purchase, usually because of scarce financial resources. Many times, neither medical nor administrative departments are included on a committee to allow a rational discussion of the advantages of acquiring new techniques, their cost-effectiveness and an analysis of the financial viability of the acquisition. Technological advances constitute a factor responsible for the rapid development of critical care medicine in the last three decades. Nevertheless, the use of technology in the intensive care context has been subjected to increasing criticism in the course of recent years from a medical, bioethics and economic point of view.

- Medical considerations: Technology being offered in the market often does not have evidence based on well-prepared studies to demonstrate its utility for patient care. There is no doubt that the incorporation of microprocessed ventilators, pulse oxymetry, capnography, measurement of intracranial pressure (ICP) and many other technologies have introduced important changes in patient management; nevertheless, it is an obligation of the ICU director to evaluate carefully new technologies or variations of already existing technology before deciding as to the benefits of its incorporation or change.

- One essential issue for deciding to add a new technology is to evaluate if the human available are able to cope with the new equipment. It is necessary to assess if the introduction of the new technology does not go against some cultural paradigm about how the task should be carried out. Education of human resources as to the advantages and results achieved with new technologies are necessary for implementing their use correctly. The necessary changes in working procedures must be done smoothly through educational programmes and must be ideally explained in written protocols that the organisation can handle easily. New procedures introduced by the incorporation of new technology not only refer to its application in patients, but also to the impact in other hospital areas, examples being engineering, sterilisation, infection prevention, etc. A third issue to be considered is that the financial viability of introducing the new technology does not only refer to the purchase process but also and mainly to the preventive maintenance and fixing of the instruments. Frequently in many countries with scarce resources, a new procedure, equipment or technology is not used because it is not possible to maintain it because of budget shortfalls for the purchase of spare parts or for correct preventive maintenance.

- Bioethics considerations: These have to do with the excessive use of resources in patients with a poor pathology or from which no recovery is possible. Many times, the patient or his family continue to demand the use of relatively complex vital support systems. It is known that the intensive care areas use enormous hospital and social resources that are lacking for other health system programmes. Deviations in the rational use of resources affect three rules of bioethics: the medical beneficence principle as stated by Hippocrates, patient autonomy rights and distributive equity. It is necessary that technology use be able to depend rational guidelines that preclude the excessive use of life support as long as possible in the case of pathological conditions from which no recovery is possible in a short time.

- Economic considerations: This has to do with the medical and financial evaluation of new technology and with the availability of financial resources. The ICU director must find out if an economic analysis of the utility of the new procedures at least has been done. This financial analysis, obviously, does not only refer to funds resources, but mainly to studies of cost-effectiveness, cost-utility and cost-benefits of the new techniques. If these studies exist and support the use of a technology, we must still remember that the conclusions of studies effected in countries with a greater degree of human and economic development and resources, cannot be mechanically extrapolated to developing or undeveloped countries. The American Society of Critical Care Medicine (SCCM) has established guides referring to technology evaluation and use (Table 4).

Table 4. Evaluation of new technology (adapted from [9])

What basic science principles support a certain technology?

Are the indications for the use of the new technology clearly indicated by the manufacturing company?

Are secondary advantages defined for frequent users?

Does the new technology really comply with the indications proposed by the manufacturing company?

Which is the scientific information available to support its use?

Is scientific information available on key concepts about the new technology?

Does this information consider: survival, morbidity, length of stay in the ICU, benefits and complications?

How high are the costs of introducing the new technology, including initial capital, operating costs, costs of human and non human resources to be used, and indirect costs?

How does the technology affect the total daily cost of the patient?

Does new technology require special trained staff, such as knowledge in basic sciences or specific experience for its safe use?

In summary, the UCI still faces considerable problems in terms of technology incorporation and use. Issues such as evaluation of appropriate new instruments and techniques, financial resources for purchase, preventive maintainance and repair, the education of human resources, changes in cultural patterns of the health team for accepting new task procedures, have still not found definitive answers around the world.

References

1. Hanson CW, Deustshman CS, Anderson HL et al (1999) Effects of organized critical care services on outcomes and resources utilization: A cohort study. Crit Care Med 27:270–274
2. Cullen DJ, Civetta JM, Briggs BA et al (1974) Therapeutic Intervention Scoring System: A method of quantitative comparison of patient care. Crit Care Med 2:57–60
3. Miranda DR , de Rijk A, Schaufeli W (1996) Simplified Therapeutic Intervention Scoring System : the TISS-28 items. Results from a multicenter study. Crit Care Med 24:64–73
4. Moreno R, Morais P (1997) Validation of the simplified therapeutic intervention scoring system on an independent database. Intensive Care Med 23:640–644
5. Miranda DR, Nap R, de Rijk A et al (2003) Nursing activities score. Crit Care Med 31:374–382
6. Weber RJ, Kane SL, Oriolo VA (2003) Impact of intensive care unit (ICU) drug use on hospital costs: A descriptive analysis, with recommendations for optimizing ICU pharmacotherapy. Crit Care Med 31:S17–S24
7. Hoffman JM, Shah ND, Vermeulen LC et al (2005) Projecting future drug expenditure. Am J Health Syst Pharm 62:149–167
8. Pierpaoli PG (1993) The rising costs of pharmaceuticals: A director of pharmacy's perspective. Am J Hosp Pharm 50:S6–S8
9. Anonymous (1993) A model for technology assessment applied to pulse oximetry. The Technology Assessment Task Force of the Society of Critical Care Medicine. Crit Care Med 21:615–624

Sepsis and Organ(s) Dysfunction – Key Points, Reflections, and Perspectives

A. Gullo, F. Iscra, F. Rubulotta

Introduction and Background

Sepsis is one of the main problems in medicine due to its complexity from pathophysiology, clinical, and therapeutic standpoints. Although several definitions have been proposed for this syndrome, it can in general be assumed that it represents the clinical manifestation of a system response of the body to infection or to an inflammatory-associated acute disease [1, 2]. Despite advances in medical practice, sepsis, severe sepsis, and septic shock, associated with different grading of organ(s) dysfunction/failure, are conditions that significantly limit quality of life and the ultimate survival of intensive care unit (ICU) patients. In any case, the health cost implications remain exorbitant [3]. Mortality rates as a result of sepsis are associated with a pattern characterized by progressive dysfunction/failure of non-pulmonary organ systems and, in particular, worsening neurologic, coagulation, and renal dysfunction over the first three days. Although initial pulmonary dysfunction is common in patients with sepsis syndrome, it is not associated with an increased mortality rate [4]. In five recent clinical trials that enrolled a total of 5661 patients with severe sepsis – the criteria being evidence of infection, systemic inflammatory response syndrome (SIRS), and at least one organ dysfunction/hypoperfusion – the incidences of septic shock ranged from 52 to 71% in the group of patients with severe sepsis. The mean was 58% [5–9]. A recent study used the International Classification of Diseases (ICD) nine hospital diagnostic codes for infection and acute organ dysfunction – to estimate 751 000 cases of severe sepsis per annum in the United States [3]. According to this data, septic shock would, therefore, be predicted to occur annually in 435 580 patients in the US. Mortality rate is a consequence of one or more factors such as: age, immunodepression, presence of diseases and/or chronic failure of one or multiple organ system dysfunctions and/or failure [10, 11]. Pathophysiologic mechanisms are basically related to Gram-negative bacteria endotoxin [12], but also Gram-positive micro-organisms, viruses, and mycetes, which are supposedly responsible for the local and systemic release of several mediators that, in turn, might be responsible for the organic response to infection, characterised by cardiovascular instability, hyperthermia, hypothermia, leukocytes, and coagulation alterations as well as by involvement of one or multiple organs [13]. The term sepsis is related to the concept of multiple organ dysfunction syndrome (MODS), which is frequently identified with the end result of infection, although it has been shown that septic syndrome is not specific to infection and can also originate as a result of a variety of non-infectious stimuli such as pancreatitis, burns, and trauma [14]. The American College of Chest Physicians proposed new definitions for sepsis and organ failure and guidelines for the use of innovative therapies in sepsis [15]. Indeed, although remarkable progress has been achieved in defining the pathophysiology of sepsis, the terminology associated with research in this field has remained confusing.

The term SIRS, which until recently was very controversial, was developed to imply a clinical response arising from a non-specific insult; it includes two or more non-specific variables. Sepsis is defined as SIRS with documented infection. The sequela of SIRS/sepsis is multiple organ dysfunction syndrome (MODS), which can be defined as the failure to maintain homeostasis without intervention. Primary MODS is a direct result of a well-defined insult, while secondary MODS develops not as a direct response to an insult, but as the consequence of a host response. Roger Bone confirmed the above problems by reporting his personal experience with SIRS [16]. Several studies that examined the risk factors leading to sepsis (Table 1) were able to predict patients' outcome: the age 65 years or older, the coexistance of chronic diseases, and the presence of surgical sepsis [17]. The Centers for Disease Control and Prevention (CDC) evidenced the risk factors for developing septic shock, such as the presence of a central catheter, parenteral nutrition, antibiotic use, the presence of an arterial catheter, or an endotracheal tube. Other risk factors found to predict the development of Gram-negative bac-

Table 1. Sepsis predisposition

- Age
- Infection
- Site of infections
- Co-morbidity
- Severity
- Gender
- Genotype
- Mediator/marker

teremia included the following: admission to an ICU, use of broad-spectrum antibiotics, immunosuppressive treatments, invasive procedures and devices, burns, trauma, advanced age, cancer, acquired immunodeficiency syndrome (AIDS), fever, low systolic blood pressure, and low platelet counts [18, 19].

Immune Inflammatory Response and Biomarkers

The immune-inflammatory process is a normal response to infection and is essential not only for the resolution of infection, but also for the initiation of other adaptive stress responses required for host survival. The profound redundancy of action of many cytokines means that there are many overlapping pathways for cellular activation and further mediator release. In addition, the synergism of actions and effects of many cytokines suggests that imbalance in the process of the immune response may be adversely affected by inhibition of a single agent. Mediators of immunity and inflammation are part of an intercellular signalling language that allows cells/tissue/organs to take in new information and, based on past experience, decide what to do next. There are essentially two components to the immune response – innate (non-specific) and acquired (antibody mediated) immunity. The complement system is a multi-component triggered enzyme cascade that attracts phagocytes to microorganisms increasing capillary permeability and neutrophil chemotaxis and adhesion. Specific-acquired immunity in the form of antibodies inactivates microorganisms that are not destroyed by the innate immune system. Such microorganisms either fail to activate the complement pathway or prevent activation of phagocytes. The cells involved in innate immunity include 'professional' phagocytes (polymorphonuclear neutrophils, mastcells, and macrophages) and 'non-professional' phagocytes (endothelial cells and hepatocytes). Cells infected with viruses and parasites are killed by large granular lymphocytes termed natural killer (NK) cells, and eosinophils. Acquired immune defences against specific micro-organisms (antigens) form the second component of the immune response. Antibodies activate the component system, stimulate phagocytic cells, and specifically inactivate microorganisms. Lymphocytes, the basis of the acquired immune defence system, consist of antibody-producing plasma cells derived from B-lymphocytes, and T-lymphocytes that control intracellular infections. Binding of microorganisms to antibodies on the cell surface of B-cells leads to preferential selection of these antibody-producing cells. This is termed priming, and subsequent responses are faster and amplified, and provide the basis of vaccination. T-cells exploit two main strategies to combat intracellular infections – the secretion of soluble mediators, which activates other cells to enhance microbial defence mechanisms and the production of cytolytic T-cells that kill the target organism. Adaptive selection of specific T-cell subsets occurs in response to local balance of cytokine concentrations [20]. Hollenberg et al. [21] reported the existence of a circulating vasodilating substance that may play a role in the pathogenesis of septic states. As the sepsis condition progresses, there is evidence of a complex disturbance in vasomotor tone (peripheral vasculopathy), characterised by non-specific systemic vasodilation, pulmonary vasoconstriction, and increased vascular permeability. Pinsky and Matuschak [22] showed that endotoxaemia in an experimental model in animals produced a marked increase of peripheral vascular capacitance without changing in compliance. Vasodilation was unrelated to the level endogenous autonomic tone. Peripheral vascular paralysis leads to the inability to regulate the distribution of blood flow to the peripheral circulation. The ominous importance of this vasculopathy was shown in a clinical study by Parker et al. [23]. Experimental and clinical studies indicated that the excess release of pro-inflammatory cytokines and other host-derived inflammatory mediators contributed to the basic pathophysiology of human septic shock [24]. Cytokines are the primary communicators of the innate immune system; they serve the body as chemical messengers between cells and are involved in such processes as cell growth and differentiation, tissue repair and remodelling, and the regulation of immune response [25]. Large quantities of TNF-α, IL-1, or many other inflammatory mediators (which are good for the host in localised infections), are detrimental when released in systemic circulation. Cytokines are a group of small signalling proteins produced by a large variety of cells that are thought to be important for host defence, wound healing, and other essential host functions. While cytokines are generally viewed as a destructive development in the patient that generally leads to multiple organ dysfunction, cytokines also protect the body when localised. Cytokines are highly pleiotropic, and they appear capable of producing markedly different effects depending on the nearby hormonal milieu. Furthermore, the body has a highly complex, tightly regulated network of receptor antagonists and other regulatory agents that continuously modulate the effects of cytokine release. This fact may explain why the trials of various anti-cytokine agents have produced disappointing results [24]. Although cytokines are important for these homeostatic functions, excessive production and release of cytokines initiate widespread tissue injury, which can result in organ dysfunction. Four cytokines, TNF-α, IL-1, IL-6 and IL-8, have been most strongly associated with sepsis syndrome. Cytokines are not stored in intracellular compartments, and are newly synthetised and released in response to inflammatory stimuli. This regulation occurs predominantly at the level of gene transcription with the new expression of cytokine mRNA. Cytokines have a synergistic, overlapping, and antagonistic effect. Anti-inflammatory cytokines, as well as pro-inflammatory cytokines, are produced following upon the activation of the cytokine cascade. The sequela of SIRS/sepsis is multiple organ dysfunction failure. This condition has been defined as the swinging of a pendulum across the whole spectrum of SIRS, compensatory anti-inflammatory response syndrome (CARS), and mixed antagonist response syndrome (MARS). Tissue insult/injury triggers a triad of systems encompassing the macrophages, cytokines, and endothelial cells. This results in SIRS/CARS/MARS, which results in terminal organ dysfunction. This condition can progress to MODS, particularly when aggravated by a second hit (another tissue insult/injury), or it can move towards resolution, particularly when second hits are avoided [26]. The interaction between pro-inflammatory and anti-inflammatory mediators can be viewed as a battle between opposing forces, which are often unbalanced. Initially, these mediators interact in the microenvironments. If the mediators balance each other and the initial response is overcome, homeostasis is restored. If they do not, pro-inflammatory and anti-inflammatory mediators may be found in systemic circulation. If balance cannot be established there and homeostasis is not restored, a massive pro-inflammatory reaction (SIRS) or an anti-inflammatory reaction (CARS) will ensue. A range of clinical sequelae may then follow in accordance with the acronym CHAOS (Table 2).

Table 2. CHAOS induced by SIRS/CARS/MARS (modified from [27])

C	Cardiovascular compromise (usually manifesting as shoch; in this setting SIRS predominates
H	Homeostasis (return to health; this represents a balance between SIRS and CARS
A	Apoptosis (programmed cell death; SIRS predominates)
O	Organ dysfunction, single or multiple anergy or increased susceptibility to infection; CARS predominates
S	Suppression of the immune system; here again, SIRS predominates

Inflammatory response is a highly orchestrated system of cellular activity and locale release of pro-inflammatory and anti-inflammatory response. The released cytokines and inflammatory mediators activate and modulate the responses of other immunocytes to attack and destroy the infecting microbes [28].

In contrast with many acute and severe diseases, such as acute myocardial infarction, pancreatitis, renal and liver failure, adrenal dysfunction etc., sepsis lacks specific markers. Several biomarkers of sepsis have been proposed, such as circulating non-segmented neutrophils, acute phase proteins such as

C-reactive protein, and neopterin, cytokines (TNF-α and IL-6), and chemokine (IL-8) [29]. Practically all of the above mentioned markers have shown some utility in detecting a septic condition, but all of them lack specificity for severe infection or for infection-inducing organ dysfunction and/or shock. Procalcitonin blood levels were first reported in 1993 in paediatric patients suffering sepsis [30]. The monitoring of procalcitonin blood levels is useful in identifying patients with severe sepsis and septic shock [31]. Procalcitonin also represents an important marker able to differentiate SIRS patients from those with sepsis [32]. However, sepsis diagnosis represents a true challenge considering the prevalence of aspecific clinical signs such as tachicardia, tachypnoea, leukocytosis, and fever. On the other hand, blood cultures from patients suffering sepsis may be positive in only 30 to 40% of cases. The exact cellular and organ source for the pro-hormone, its regulation, and its relationship with bacteria and bacterial products remains largely unknown [29]. The prognostic value of daily measurements of procalcitonin appears superior to that of C-reactive protein [33].

Microcirculation Dysfunction

Microcirculatory dysfunction during sepsis is not the consequence of one single metabolic or other defect or of one single mediator – even though TNF-α and IL-1β have long been explored as central mediators in sepsis – but of a rather complex, still not completely understood cascade of mediators. The coagulation cascade and the complement system become activated, and arachidonic acid is metabolised to form leukotrienes, thromboxane, and prostaglandins. T-cells are activated to release cytokines and growth stimulatory factors. Most of these mediator systems affect the microcirculation in one or more ways, and there is a striking redundancy in their modes of action. For instance, endotoxin, TNF-α, PAF, and leukotrienes have all been shown to affect the endothelial barrier function individually, and it can be speculated how they might act in concert to damage circulation during sepsis [34].

Systemic inflammation, which occurs during sepsis, leads to a complex biological interaction with profound changes in endothelial function [35]. The endothelium itself may release nitric oxide or endothelin, with antagonistic effects on vascular tone. Many mediators, including complement fragments, may either prime and/or directly stimulate neutrophils to release inflammatory mediators, reactive oxygen species, or hydrolytic enzymes, to aggregate with each other and or platelets, to adhere to endothelial cells, and finally to obstruct capillary lumina. Further players in the above mediator cascade include kallikrein, kinins, thrombin, endorphins, and heat-shock proteins. Maintenance of optimal tissue perfusion is important to minimise ischaemia-induced cellular injury and to decrease ischaemia resulting from stress and the inflammatory response. Inadequate oxygen supply to tissues relative to cellular consumption results in an oxygen debt that impairs cellular function. The vasopressor and inotropic agents, in particular epinephrine and dobutamine, have been shown to exert vasodilatory effects on the gastric microcirculation as assessed by a laser Doppler flowmetry, and thereby improve oxygen delivery to splanchnic organs [36]. Nitric oxide is a potent vasodilator at the microcirculatory level [37] and alters microvascular permeability. In clinical trials with septic patients, the inhibition of nitric oxide yielded increases in blood pressure, but at the same time showed increases in liver enzymes and increased pulmonary resistance evidencing the jeopardised microvascular blood flow and tissue oxygenation [38].

Experimental and clinical trials have demonstrated positive effects of hypertonic fluids in patients with sepsis-related ARDS, and found significant increases in systemic and pulmonary arterial pressure, increased cardiac output, increased stroke volumes and, at the same time, significant improvements in tissue oxygen delivery and consumption. One of the novel approaches to treating sepsis is to intervene at specific key events within the signal transduction cascade. It becomes increasingly evident that the transcription factor NF-kB is one of the principal final common pathways in regulating genes participating in immune and inflammatory responses, including numerous genes encoding cytokines, growth factors, ICAM, and acute phase proteins [39]. How NF-kB activation can be limited within the context of MODS and sepsis is being considered at this time as a possible target for therapeutic intervention [40]. To date, therapeutic approaches such as anticytokine and anti-oxidant regimens, which have been highly successful in experimental models, have failed to demonstrate clinical efficacy.

Coagulation Pathways

Activation of the coagulation system assumes a key role in septic patients. The key role of the inflammatory response of microvascular endothelium on the progress of organ dysfunction is a well known process. In fact, it is true that Factor Xa induces the expression of a range of inflammatory cytokines such as interleukin 6 (IL-6) and IL-8 as well as adhesion molecules in endothelial cells in culture [41].

Clinical experience evidenced an activation of clotting factors and endogenous anticoagulants such as anti-thrombin III and protein C. In spite of this, a condition of disseminated intravascular coagulation (DIC) in sepsis is very seldom seen except in some specific situations such as meningococcal septicaemia. In experimental and clinical studies of sepsis it has been demonstrated that fibrin deposition in several organs and the subsequent activation of fibrinolysis may be an important protective mechanism preventing MODS in patients with DIC [42, 43]. The inflammatory response flowing exposure to lipopolysaccharide (LPS) or tumour necrosis factor (TNF) is one example. It is known that F expression is regulated by activator protein 1 (AP 1) and nuclear factor kB (NF-kB), two transcription factors known to regulate other mediators of inflammation [44]. The inhibition of the TF/Factor VIIa pathways in animal experiments through the administration of monoclonal antibodies showed no evidence of DIC following infusion of endotoxin or live Escherichia coli [45].

The physiological regulatory mechanisms of coagulation impaired by activation of coagulation cascade may contribute to fibrin formation. Plasma levels of the most important inhibitor of thrombin, ATIII, are usually markedly reduced in sepsis. This is a consequence of a combination of increased consumption, degradation by elastase released from activated neutrophils, and also impaired synthesis.

In addition, there is a decrease in the protein C/protein S system that also enhances the pro-coagulation state [46]. Protein C is a circulating protein that is an inactive precursor of protease and is converted to APC in the presence of the thrombin/thrombomodulin complex. There is a protein C receptor, called endothelial protein C receptor, which facilitates activation of protein C; however, it is not an absolute requirement for activation. APC inactivated Factors Va and VIIIa limit thrombin generation [47] and also promote fibrinolysis by inhibiting activity of the plasminogen activator inhibitor 1 [48]. It is also suggested that APC may reduce inflammation by inhibiting cytokine production and white cell activation [49]. APC was shown to have a protective role against MODS and mortality in experimental models of sepsis [50] and has subsequently been shown to decrease mortality in human beings suffering severe sepsis [7].

Early Source Control

The early localisation of infection is crucial for the clinical evolution of sepsis; abdominal sepsis means synonymous of peritonitis. Abdominal sepsis is classified as primary, secondary, and tertiary.

Primary peritonitis is characterised by spontaneous bacterial peritonitis or catheter infections.

Secondary peritonitis is from perforations and anastomotic leaks, pancreatitis, cholecystitis, and similar conditions. In tertiary peritonitis there might be a marked inflammatory response in the abdomen without pathogenesis or with only low-grade pathogens that usually occurs after control of the secondary or primary insult. Frequently, the patient suffers from an occult abdomen-borne sepsis, a condition that can be accompanied by changes in mental functions and disorders affecting one or more organs. In some circumstances, the main issue is the difficulty in determining whether the abdominal situation is a secondary factor to the septic process. Necrotic tissue identification can be difficult, especially in the event of deep infections [51].

Moreover, antibiotic treatments are often administered in an empirical manner, even though this approach can turn out to be effective, given that patients who are administered antibiotics show a better survival rate [52] than those not treated with antibiotics. At any rate, when bacteriological data is available, the choice of antibiotic treatments should be goal-directed. Under these circumstances, single antibiotic treatments can be as effective as combined antibiotic treatments [53, 54].

However, most comparative studies about the choice of antibiotic treatments were performed on neutropenic patients. Therefore, the comparison between these findings and those relative to a population of patients affected by severe sepsis is not justified [55].

Improved diagnostic imaging, sonography, and CT scanning in particular have paved the way for more accurate and timely diagnosis, and prognosis has consequently improved. Besides, frequently, percutaneous drainage is the method of choice in the majority of abdominal abscesses in high-risk patients, while surgery is preferred for the treatment of deep abscesses, which are difficult to remove with lower invasive techniques.

Scoring Systems and PIRO Model

Scoring systems as a means of mortality risk/severity of illness prediction have evolved from the simple identification of risk factors in an attempt to summarise and quantify these individual findings.

Several scores, such as the APACHE II (age, physiology, chronic health evaluation) and the SAPS II (simplified acute physiology score) are not satisfactory defining organ failure. Several scores recently developed, e.g. MODS (multiple organ dysfunction score), SOFA (sepsis-related organ failure assessment), choose to study the following six organs: respiratory, renal, haematologic, liver, cardiovascular, and neurologic.

It is accepted that the degree of gastrointestinal dysfunction would be useful to quantitate, particularly with recent experimental and clinical data, in its role in the pathogenesis of MOF. Unfortunately, accurate assessment of gastrointestinal function is still virtually impossible (Table 3).

Table 3. Scoring systems

Organ System	Measurable parameters
Respiratory	PaO_2/FiO_2
Renal	Serum creatinine
Haematologic	Platelet count
Central nervous	Glasgow coma score
Hepatic	Serum bilirubine
Cardiovascular	Blood pressure
Gastrointestinal	No appropriate one

A working group of the European Society of Intensive Care Medicine developed recently the SOFA score. In contrast to older scores, the aim of the SOFA score is not to predict outcome but to describe organ dysfunction. SOFA studies six organs with a scale for each from 0 (normal) to 4 (worse situation), using parameters readily available and routinely measured in most ICUs (Table 4).

The use of such scoring systems alone cannot guide acute changes in therapy but the regular, daily calculation of scores can provide an objective assessment of the evolution of the disease process and the response to therapy. They can also be employed to facilitate stratification of patients and comparison of results in clinical trials of new therapies. Considering the complexity of the septic process and to facilitate patients' enrollment in the clinical trials, several researchers have suggested the introduction in the clinical practice of a sort of cancer scoring system, since this situation is assimilable to a sepsis condition.

The PIRO model has been introduced to define septic patients [56, 57], starting with the concept of several similarities existing between sepsis and cancer: intricated pathophysiolgy, high indices of mortality, organs and system involvement, different medical and surgical management strategies, and the high cost of combined pharmacological treatment. PIRO definition describes different aspects related to sepsis: Predisposition, Infection, the host Response, and Organ(s) dysfunction/failure. Predisposition (P) factors assume a key role of individual genetic characterisation during health conditions or during the disease process such as ageing, chronic illness, or immunesuppression related to a chronic pharmacological management, etc. Recent advances in the genetic characterisation techniques evidenced the importance of knowing the several factors able to increase the risk of infection and the mortality index as a consequence of sepsis. TNFa genetic polymorphism and TNF-2 allel polymorphism induce a high blood level of

Table 4. SOFA score

SOFA score	1	2	3	4
Lung PaO_2/FiO_2 (mmHg)	< 400	< 300	< 200	< 100
Coagulation Platelets X10/mm3	≤ 150	≤ 100	≤ 50	≤ 20
Liver, Bilirubine mg/dl	1.2-1.9	2.0-5.9	6.0-11.9	12
Cardiovascolar Hypotension*	MAP	Dopamine ≤ 5 µKg/min Dobutamine ≥ 2-4µKg/min	Dopamine ≥ 5 µKg/min Epinefrine ≥ 0.1µKg/min Norepinefrine ≥ 0.1µKg/min	Dopamine ≥ 1.5 µKg/min Epinefrine ≥ 0.1µKg/min Norepinefrine ≥ 0.1µKg/min
Central Nervous System GCS	13-14	10-12	6-9	≤ 6
Kidney Creatinine, mg/dl	1.2-1.9	2.0-3.4	3.5-4.9	
Mmol/L Diuresis	(110-170)	(171-299)	(300-440) o (500ml/die)	440 o 220ml/die

* adrenergetic agents infusion more than 1 hour with the dosage of µKg/min

TNF with an increased mortality rate during septic shock [58]. Infection (I) is the second key point causing host response and decision making for the treatment. This condition includes several elements such as: bacteria type; infection localisation; and, for example, urinary tract infection vs. pulmonary infection; and the seriousness of the infection such as lobar pneumonia vs. bilateral pneumonia etc.

Response (R) is the third element. This term means the host's capacity to react to the septic; this condition may be validated in the presence of other important signs such as the number of white cells, protein C, and the procalcitonin blood level etc. Organ (O) dysfunction is the last element in the PIRO model. Created by the European Society of Intensive Care [59], the SOFA score is a good index (Table 4) to use to establish the severity of organ dysfunction, although the final score expresses the level of morbidity rather than the mortality index. It represents an important sequential index to evaluate entity of organ dysfunction [60] or the improvement of clinical conditions.

Early Goal Directed Therapy (EGDT) and Standards of Care

Lundberg et al. [61] reported that, with reference to hospitalised patients affected by septic shock, there were significant delays in the decision to transfer these patients to ICUs. They also reported that delaying the administration of fluid therapies and inotropic drugs has a huge impact on the increase in mortality rates.

Rivers et al. [9] reported that early aggressive therapy before admission to ICUs in order to treat patients affected by severe sepsis and septic shocks significantly reduced mortality. The same study also proved that decreases in morbidity and mortality rates depended on early identification and treatment of at-risk patients. Therefore, it is crucial to adopt an early approach when patients are admitted to emergency departments [62], and have this approach be facilitated by the presence of experienced teams, as well as by the possibility to pose early diagnosis and to assess the patients' disease severity by means of commonly known severity indicators used for patients in ICUs (APACHE II, SAPS II, SOFA). In particular, the early use of procalcitonin [63] and C-reactive protein values, as well as the dosage of inflammation mediators, can be very useful in making an early diagnosis of sepsis. These simple diagnostic tests can be combined with non-invasive haemodynamic methods and mixed venous blood saturation monitoring, whereas sublingual capnography can show the impairment degree of haemodynamic values [64] and early control of glycaemia value represents an important standard of care [65]. However, several supportive measures are necessary to optimise the standards of care such as: patients' posture during artificial ventilation, central venous catheterisation aseptic manoeuvres, hand washing to manage each patient, timing and selection of antibiotics, prevention of nosocomial infection for patients at risk, stress ulcer prevention, thoracic drainages when indicated for infection control, support ventilation techniques using low tidal volume and protective manoeuvres, and protocol of sedation and analgesia. Preserving tissue oxygenation and function is a priority when treating sepsis. Optimising the treatment of septic patients is based on some key factors: suppression of the focus of infection, goal-directed antibiotic treatment [66, 67], and aggressive shock treatment [68–75]. Taking into account that the old dispute about crystalloids-colloids does not lead to positive results on the prevalence of first approach on the second one on the contrary, with reference to vasopressing agents, dopamine remains the preferred drug, although epinephrine, norepinephrine, phenylephrine, and vasopressin are effective in order to improve arterial pressure and haemodynamics in patients affected by septic shock [71]. Aggressive treatments can be decisive. In this context, it is very interesting to read the recent contribution by Rivers et al. [9], who reported that early optimisation of haemodynamics can significantly reduce mortality in the event of sepsis. In particular, this study was aimed at assessing whether early circulation support before admission to ICUs of patients affected by sepsis could lead to decreases in morbidity and mortality rates. The authors enrolled 263 patients with suspected infection and SIRS signs, lactacidaemia levels higher than 4mM/L, or systolic pressure lower than 90 mmHg after proper resuscitation manoeuvres. Patients were recruited within one hour of their arrival at the hospital. The intensive care unit team that received the patients was not aware of the random assignment of patients to the various groups. Central venous pressure, average arterial pressure and hourly diuresis were measured every hour. The patients assigned to early treatment protocol were also controlled for SvO_2. When the SvO_2 value was below 70mmHg, blood transfusions were performed in order to obtain a haemoglobin concentration of 10 g/dl. For patients who reached this value, but whose SvO_2 value remained low, an infusion of 20 mcg/kg/min of dobutamine was given, and this treatment was not discontinued during intensive care. The patients, divided into two groups, were uniformly distributed by sex and age. All patients were compulsorily followed up by the emergency department for at least six hours, whereas the patients belonging to the control group were admitted to the ICU when the first bed became available. The analysis of the results obtained from both groups of patients showed that they achieved the objective of average arterial pressure and central venous pressure value optimisation within six hours. However, 40% of the patients belonging to the control group failed to reach SvO_2 values of 70%. The check of resuscitation endpoints after 72 hours showed a lasting positive effect for patients who were administered haemodynamic support with reference to both their haemodynamic indicator and organ dysfunction level. Intra-hospital mortality was 16% lower and statistically significant (P = 0.009) in patients submitted to the early-goal directed therapy in comparison with the control group (46.5% vs. 30%). This difference had not changed by day 28 and, although it was statistically low, it remained significantly better after 60 days (P = 0.03).

Clinical Trials and Human Recombinant Activated Protein C (rhAPC)

Despite the medical advances made in the knowledge of inflammatory process feeding mechanisms in the course of sepsis, the findings of many clinical trials performed during the last decade have reported negative results in terms of survival. In particular, randomised and controlled studies performed with the so-called 'immunomodulating' agents have not shown any improvements in the survival rates. Why did these studies fail? There are many explanations, such as unsuitable laboratory data or ineffective experimental agents (for instance, anti-endotoxin, HA-1 and E5). As a matter of fact, researchers thought that these agents could bind to the lipid A portion of endotoxin and hence, neutralise endotoxin activity, whereas in vitro tests proved that none of these compounds could limit endotoxin activity or reduce interleukin (IL-1) or tumour necrosis factor (TNF-α) releases [76]. Protein C plays an important role in maintaining coagulation homeostasis. Infact, in the course of sepsis, protein C levels decrease, whereas endothelial injuries weaken protein C functions, since they reduce its activation. Moreover, low protein C levels are quite frequently reported for patients affected by sepsis and septic shock. This factor plays a decisive role in the coagulation process and has important anti-inflammatory functions, including the ability to stop nuclear translocation NF-kB factor [77], which is a key mechanism for cytokine formation from mononucleate cells and endothelium. In this context, activated protein C is likely to modulate an anti-apoptosis action and to limit endothelial injuries. Protein C is a Vit K-dependant protease; protein C is converted into activated protein C when thrombin combines with thrombomodulin, a trans-membrane glycoprotein factor contained in endothelium. Activated protein C inhibits Va and VIIa factors, thus actually reducing thrombin production. Moreover, it modulates endogenous fibrinolytic activity and inflammatory response. The fast protein C depletion in the event of sepsis induces, together with other factors, coagulopathy, which leads to a severe prognosis. The decrease in thrombomodulin levels in the blood of patients suffering from meningococcaemia suggests that the ability to convert protein C into activated protein C is impaired. On the contrary, soluble thrombomodulin can stop the formation of clots and cell activation. Moreover, protein C activation and the ability to inhibit thrombin in various experimental models suggests that soluble thrombomodulin can be useful for treating sepsis. Only activated protein C, and not protein C, showed a low decrease in mortality at both the experimental and clinical levels [78]. The safety and effectiveness of human recombinant activated protein C (Drotrecogin-α) for severe sepsis treatment was demonstrated by a recent multicentre stage III trial in which 1690 patients affected by severe sepsis were enrolled [7]; as for patients treated with APC, a decrease in mortality rates down to 24.7% was reported compared with the placebo group, which recorded a mortality of 30.8%. Drotrecogin α was administered at a dosage of 24μ/kg/hour x 96 hours. In this study, the incidence of severe bleeding was higher for the group treated with APC than for the control group (3.5% vs. 2.0 %).

Selective Digestive Decontamination (SDD)

The optimal management of severe sepsis and septic shock is complex and represents a real challenge. The authors of the Surviving Sepsis Campaign selected several interventions, including bicarbonate therapy, deep venous thrombosis prophylaxis, and considerations for limitation of support. Currently, there have been five evidence-based medicine manoeuvres showing a survival benefit in ICU patients (Table 5). Only one manoeuvre is supported by at least two level 1 investigations, providing level 1 evidence with grade A recommendation, and that is selective decontamination of the digestive tract (SDD) [79]. The other four are supported by only one trial, providing a grade B recommendation [80–82]. SDD can be administered to all patients at risk of infection, whereas the other four can only be administered in specific subsets of ICU patients. It is difficult to understand the reason for omission of SDD intervention in the Surviving Sepsis Campaign guidelines, despite the availability of 54 randomised, controlled trials with seven meta-analysis showing a significant reduction of infectious morbidity and mortality [83]. The rationale behind the manoeuvre of SDD is the observation that critically ill patients develop infection with their own gut microorganisms, and that enteral antimicrobials in combination with early administration of parenteral antibiotics improve survival in critically ill patients [84]. A major difference between the only parenteral antibiotic used and SDD is that enteral antibiotics also impact the flora of the oropharynx and gut, whereas systemic agents only treat the lungs, blood, and bladder.

Table 5. Intensive care unit interventions that reduce mortality

Intervention	Relative Risk (95% CI)	Absolute Mortality Reduction % (95% CI)	No. needed to treat
Low tidal volume [80]	0.78 (0.65-0.93)	8.8(2.4-15.3)	11
Activated protein C [7]	0.80 (0.69-0.94)	6.1(1.9-10.4)	16
Intensive insulin [65]	0.44 (0.36-0.81)	3.7 (1.3-6)	27
< 5 days	0.52 (0.33-0.84)	9.6 (3-16.1)	10
Steroids [84]	0.90 (0.74-1.09)	6.4 (-4.8-17.6)	16
Non responders	0.83 (0.66-1-04)	10.8 (-1.9-23.6)	9
Selective decontamination [82]	0.65 (0.49-0.85)	8.1 (3.1-13)	12

Steroids

In 1980, Roger Bone et al. [77] performed a study aimed at demonstrating that corticosteroid administration could suppress inflammatory response thanks to its ability to modulate signal transmission at the cell level.

In particular, the anti-inflammatory role of corticosteroids was demonstrated with reference to the following aspects: ability to prevent inflammatory cascade activation by the complement, possibility to inhibit endotoxin-induced leukocyte adhesion, assessment of endotoxinaemia-induced platelet factor activation level, assessment of tumour necrosis factor and interleukin-1 releases by monocytes, and prevention of prostaglandin production through phospholipase A2 inhibitor induction. Due to these elements, corticosteroids were regarded as useful in the treatment of sepsis and were able to reduce morbidity and mortality rates. However, this issue still raises many controversial points, since some physicians maintain that corticosteroids can also be dangerous to a patient's outcome [78, 85]. Annane et al. [86] started from the assumption that absolute adrenal failure is present in about 1 to 2% of patients admitted to ICUs, whereas adrenal dysfunction occurs in 30% of patients hospitalised in the same structure. 297 patients with septic shock and dependent on vasopressors agents were enrolled. They underwent ACTH stimulation at the onset of shock and were randomly assigned hydrocortisone or fludrocortisone vs. placebo administration for seven days; the intravenous cortisone dosage was 50 mg four times a day. A significant decrease in mortality (10%) was reported in the treated patients [86, 87] compared with the control groups. These findings, although promising, are not conclusive. The stratification of at-risk patients under intensive care is a key point in daily clinical practice.

Experimental Therapies

In this context, IgM immunoglobulins seem to play an important role. As a matter of fact, a decrease in mortality and the absence of adverse effects shown with this treatment were encouraging results. In particular, immunoglobulins have various important functions such as decrease in body temperature and inflammatory parameters (procalcitonin), reduction in FiO_2 (which is an indirect sign of better oxygen saturation), and stabilisation of average arterial pressure and heart rate [88, 89]. Pentaglobin is likely to reduce morbidity and mortality in septic patients and plays an important role in immunity system modulation [90]. Of course, there are no magic wands to treat sepsis; however, in the light of the results obtained from these experimental therapies, the rationale of associating different drugs should be supported. There is increasing evidence that adenoceptor modulation can prevent tissue injury through a variety of pathways [91].

Adenosine is a metabolite of adenosine triphosphate (ATP) with a short half-life [92] due to its rapid metabolism. It accumulates in areas where ATP is used, but not reformed, such as during ischaemia [93] and possibly during sepsis [94]. Adenosine acts on a variety of cells including myocytes (AV nodal block), mast cells, macrophages, and neutrophils. There are four adenoceptors, known as A1, A2a, A2B, and A3 receptors. Endogenously released adenosine was shown to protect human vascular endothelial cells from injury by stimulated neutrophils [95]. The use of adenosine modulation in ischaemia/reperfusion injury has been the subject of considerable investigation, although experience with its use in sepsis is limited. Adenosine may attenuate I/R injury through a number of possible mechanisms [96], including purine salvaging, improved tissue perfusion, anti-inflammatory action, and a direct intracellular initiator/effector mechanism; experimental data in sepsis evidenced that adenosine strongly inhibits extracellular superoxide anion release [97]. Furthermore, adenosine has unwanted cardiovascular side effects, causing bradycardia and hypotension. Alternatives to adenosine administration include modulation of its metabolism and the administration of specific antagonists/antagonists [98].

Injury and Sepsis: Genomics and Proteinomics Perspectives

A predisposition to sepsis represents an increased risk of developing sepsis. Genetic predisposition can be considered in terms of high risk and low-risk exposure and independent and dependent exposure. High risk often involves dependence on single genes, so single mutation produces the disease, while lower risk often reflects a dependence on multiple genes. Sepsis probably is a multiple-gene problem. Acquired factors are complex and difficult to separate from heritable factors. Age, gender, chronic health or disease, acute illness, exposures, and interventions all are acquired factors. Such acquired factors confound all studies of genetic predisposition of multifactorial diseases and multidimensional responses. However, traditional genetic studies are not possible in sepsis because family members usually do not become septic at the same time and because the treatment changes over time. The study of injury in critical illness is now occurring 'upstream', at the genetic and cellular levels, to understand how damaging effects of acute inflammation from injury can be prevented or modulated. Genomic and proteinomics evidence documents that repair processes begin shortly after injury [99]. The interactions between the injury and repair cascades most likely determine the outcome of the injurious process. With closer examination of the heterogeneity inherent in the human population, the different genotypic expressions also include differences in the kind of repair response mounted. These differences include varied Th1 vs. Th2, or hyperinflammatory vs. hypoinflammatory, helper T-cell responses to a septic or inflammatory insult. In addition, different degrees of apoptosis occur, with often deleterious sequelae [100]. Definitions of injury and repair are important because they are somewhat arbitrary and may in fact be interchangeable in terms of body processes. Injury is defined as the disruption of molecular, cellular, or organ functions resulting from an external or internal stimulus. The external stimuli include infection, hypoxia, ischaemia, chemical or thermal injury, toxins, and trauma. The internal stimuli include the acute inflammation cascade, shock, and reperfusion injury. An alternative organisation groups the injurious stimuli as physical (radiation, extreme temperature, mechanical trauma), chemical (toxins), biological (infections, cell-mediated toxicity, cytokine mediated toxicity, enzymatic activity), and substrate deficiency (oxygen, glucose). Whatever the initial stimulus, once the injury occurs, they manifest similar results once the body activates its repair response. Repair is defined as an adaptive process that occurs in response to injury and involves both local and systemic responses that serve to restore structure and regulation for the purpose of organ/tissue function. The repair responses to injury probably vary as a result of genetic factors; some people react with a more vigorous inflammatory response than others [101]. They represent an organised effort to reestablish cellular and tissue integrity after injury and involve a complex order of cellular and biochemical events. The initial steps of the acute phase response include coagulation, leukocytes activation, edema formation from extravasation, and apoptosis [102].

The apoptotic response correlates with a worse outcome [103], because it can induce cell injury and death to an extent that exacerbates the morbidity of the injury [104]. Potential signals rush into and out of cells through plasma membrane disruptions. These might trigger cell or tissue level adaptive responses serving to facilitate future disruption repair or mechanically reinforce the cells environment. One well-characterised example of a signal that exists through a disruption is a fibroblast growth factor (FGF)-2. This polypeptide growth factor, like several others, lacks a signal peptide sequence and so cannot be secreted by the conventional exocytotic pathway [105]. Other repair processes include proliferation, regeneration, remodelling, revascularisation, and scar formation. Also involved in the dynamics of injury and repair are heat-shock proteins, which can be manipulated to alter the outcome of injury and repair mechanisms. The heat-shock proteins have both positive and negative effects on cytokine expression, and they modulate the tendency towards apoptosis and necrosis in stressful conditions, such as ischaemia [106] The preliminary theories of the tissue repair process, then, are compatible with the biochemical events seen in vitro. However, when applying the principles to an in vivo situation, questions still remain.

For example, with repair processes, the outcome of each organ differs. Is that a result of different repair processes occurring in the different organ system? Is the process of repair the same given different underlying mechanisms of injury – sepsis, acute respiratory distress syndrome, blunt trauma, or hemorrhagic shock? And do the differing mechanisms modify the repair process? What organs are capable of regeneration? What is the timeline of the injury and repair? Do factors such as genomics or nutritional status modulate the repair rate? These are some of the questions which require answers from researchers and clinicians in the future.

Reflections and Conclusions

In spite of the advances in the knowledge of the basic phenomenon of inflammation and its continuum for development of sepsis and organ(s) dysfunction, the search for a 'magic bullet' to treat sepsis has been frustrating. Negative clinical results for survival rates are substantially different from experimental data. Monoclonal antibody, anti-inflammatory drugs, immunoglobulins, anti-endotoxin and other aspecific therapy all failed to improve the patient's outcome as defined by the traditional primary endpoint of mortality [107].

Clinical trials remain the most effective means for assessing efficacy and safety of new therapies of sepsis [108]. After two decades of failure it is time do reconsider the target for treatment in human beings and to find a more appropriate endpoint in the treatment of sepsis. Several thousands of patients have been enrolled in the sepsis trials series managed in the past 15 years. These trials have been conducted in ICUs in heterogeneous patient population with various entry criteria and endpoints of response [107]. So, the history of the therapeutic trials in sepsis has been one of unfulfilled expectations and conflicting results until the last successful trial on Activated Protein C [7]. Sepsis is a disease, but more frequently it has become difficult to correctly define so it remains a syndrome. The development of organ dysfunction, with the signs and symptoms of sepsis and an infection, defines severe sepsis. The development of arterial hypotension in addition to organ dysfunction and symptoms of sepsis is defined as septic shock [108]. Why have all clinical trials failed? This is a question of paramount importance and must be cleared up. In fact, heterogeneity of a studied population is a crucial point; sepsis often presents with various co-morbid disease states and septic patients often receive different treatment for these co-morbid diseases. The admission diagnosis and the consistency of underlying disease remain the major determinants of outcome [109]. Scoring systems are useful to focus the relative risk of death, although the degree of organ dysfunction and even the quality of life are also important [110, 111]. Considering the poor knowledge of sepsis pathophysiology the criteria used for the patients enrolment in sepsis studies is crucial to permit the right treatment at the right time in the right group of patients. Therefore, it is important to consider the presence and the source of infection, the type of micro-organism, the severity of the underlying disease, and the appropriateness of the non-trial study therapy. Furthermore, mixing together septic patients with and without documented infections may obscure relevant therapeutic effects of the intervention tested [112].

Several aspects must be elucidated to further clarify the complexity of sepsis and related conditions. For example, considering the difficulties in having an appropriate standard of care between various institutions in multi-centre trials, it is not surprising that the outcome will differ between ICUs. Sepsis is a condition with high-consuming resources, but until now the mortality rate was not a rare event. In the clinical trials of sepsis, 28 or 30 day all cause mortality has the primary endpoint for efficacy. All cause mortality ranges between 20 and 60% and represent the overall death rate of a cohort of patients who developed bacteremic sepsis during their ICU or hospital stay [108]. In critically ill patients, the underlying disease and the functional health status are the most important determinants of outcome. Underlying disease during Gram-negative bacteraemia is the most important determinant of outcome. Thus, one may expect any novel therapeutic intervention to have only a modest effect on the outcome from severe sepsis [113].

Considering the significant cons of mortality as the primary endpoint in sepsis it has been suggested that one should not use cause mortality (28-day window) or attributable mortality as the sole endpoints, but should instead regard the reduction of reversal of organ failure as a valid efficacy endpoint (such as quality of life), which is an important parameter [114]. Starting with these observations, the importance of surrogate as an alternative to mortality has been considered. Organ failure scores represent a surrogate outcome in phase II and phase III clinical trials. Although mortality as an endpoint is characterised by some advantages, it must not be forgotten that the goal of sepsis treatment is to preserve or improve organ function. Thus, the assessment of reduction in morbidity rather than in mortality gives some advantages; five organ failure descriptors have been shown to correlate with ICU mortality in a dose-dependent fashion as does hypotension [115]. Up-to-date therapeutic interventions and target for sepsis remain a true challenge [116, 117].

References

1. Beal AL, Cerra FB (1994) Multiple organ failure syndrome in the 1990s: systemic inflammatory response and organ dysfunction. JAMA 271:226–233
2. Vincent JL, Bihari D (1992) Sepsis, severe sepsis or sepsis syndrome: need for clarification. Int Care Med 18:255–257
3. Angus DC, Linde-Zwirble WT, Lidicker J et al (2001) Epidemiology of severe sepsis

in the United States: analysis of incidence, outcome, and associated costs of care. Crit Care Med 29:1303–1310

4. Russell JA, Singer J, Bernard GR et al (2000) Changing pattern of organ dysfunction in early human sepsis is related to mortality. Crit Care Med 10:3405–3411

5. Opal SM, Fisher CJ Jr, Dhainaut JF et al (1997) Confirmatory Interleukin-1 receptor antagonist trial in severe sepsis. A phase III, randomized, double blind, placebo-controlled, multicenter trial. Crit Care Med 25:1115–1124

6. Pittet D, Hrbarth S, Suter PM et al (1999) Efficacy and safety of recombinant human activated protein C for severe sepsis. Am J Respir Crit Care Med 160:852–857

7. Bernard G, Vincent JL, Laterre PF et al (2001) Efficacy and safety of humans rhAPC for severe sepsis. N Engl J med 344:749–762

8. Warren BL, Eid A, Singer P et al (2001) Caring for the critically ill patient. High–dose antithrombin III in severe sepsis: A randomised controlled trial. JAMA 2896:1869–1878

9. Rivers E, Nguyen B, Havstad S et al (2001) Early goal-directed therapy in the treatment of severe sepsis and septic shock. N Engl J Med 345:1368–1377

10. Tran DD, Groenvald ABJ, van der Meulen J et al (1990) Age, chronic disease, sepsis, organ system failure, and mortality in a medical intensive care unit. Crit Care Med 18:474–479

11. Bone RC (1993) The systemic inflammatory response syndrome (SIRS). In: Gullo A (ed) Anesthesia, Pain, Intensive Care and Emergency (A.P.I.C.E.). Springer, Milan pp 561–571

12. Danner RL, Elin RJ, Hosseini JM et al (1991) Endotoxemia in human septic shock. Chest 99:169–175

13. Deitch EA (1992) Multiple Organ Failure: pathophysiology and potential future therapy. Ann Surg 216:117–134

14. Allardyce DB (1987) Incidence of necrotizing pancreatitis and factors related to mortality. Am J Surg 216:117–134

15. Anonymous (1992) American College of Chest Physicians/Society of Critical Care Medicine Consensus Conference: definitions for sepsis and organ failure and guidelines for the use of innovative therapies in sepsis. Crit Care Med 20(6):864–874

16. Bone RC (1996) A personal experience with SIRS and MODS. Crit Care Med 24:1417–1418

17. Heard So, Fink MP (1991) Multiple organ failure syndrome: Part1: epidemiology, prognosis and pathophysiology. J Intens Care Med 6:279–294

18. Anonymous (1993) Centers for Disease Control and Prevention. National Center for Health Statistics: Mortality Patterns – United States, 1990. Monthly Vital Statistics Report 41:45

19. Parker MM, Parrillo JE (1983) Septic Shock: Hemodynamics and pathogenesis. JAMA 250:3324–3327

20. Kuchroo VK, Das MP, Browun JA et al (1995) B7-1 and B7-2 co-stimulatory molecules activate differentially the Th1/Th2 developmental pathways. Cell 80:707–718

21. Hollenberg SM, Cunnion RE, Parrillo JE (1992) Effect of septic serum on vascular smooth muscle: in vitro studies using aortic rings. Crit Care Med 20:993–998

22. Pinsky MR, Matuschak GM (1986) Cardiovascular determinants of the hemodynamic response to acute endotoxemia in the dog. J Crit Care 1:18–31

23. Parker M, Shelhamer JH Bacharach S et al (1984) Profound but reversible myocardial depression in patients with septic shock. Ann Intern Med 100:483–490

24. Bone RC (1996) Toward a theory regarding the pathogenesis of the systemic inflammatory response syndrome: what we do and do not know about cytokine regulation. Crit Care Med 24:163–172

25. Oberholzer A, Oberholzer C, Moldawer LL (2000) Cytokine signalling - regulation of the immune response in normal and critically ill states. Crit Care Med 28:N3–N12

26. Bone RC (1996) Sir Isaac Newton, Sepsis, SIRS, and CARS. Crit Care Med 24:1125–1128

27. Bone RC (1996) Toward a theory regarding the pathogenesis of the systemic inflammatory response syndrome: what we do and do no know about cytokine regulation. Crit Care Med 24:163–172

28. Reed RL (2000) Contemporary issues with bacterial infection in the intensive care unit. Surg Clin North Am 80(3):895–909

29. Ruokonen E, Ilkka L, Niskanen M et al (2002) Procalcitonin and neopterin as indicators of infection inn critically ill patients. Acta Anaesthesiol Scand 46:398–404

30. Assicot M, Gendrel D, Carsin H et al (1993) High serum procalcitonin concentrations in patients with sepsis and infection. Lancet 341:515–518

31. Giamarellos-Bourboulis EJ, Mega A, Grecka P et al () Procalcitonin: a marker to clearly differentiate systemic inflammatory response syndrome and sepsis in the critically ill patient? Intensive Care Med 2002 Sep; 28(9):1351–1356

32. Ugarte H, Silva E, Mercan D et al (1999)Procalcitonin used as a marker of infection in the intensive care unit. Crit Care Med Mar 27(3):498–504

33. Claeys R, Vinken S, Spapen H et al (2002) Plasma procalcitonin and C-reactive protein in acute septic shock: clinical and biological correlates. Crit Care Med 30:757–762

34. Kirkpatrick CJ, Bittinger F, Klein CL et al (1996) The role of the microcirculation in multiple organ dysfunction syndrome (MODS): a review and perspectives. Virchows Arch 427:461–476

35. Reinhart K, Bayer O, Brunkhorst F et al (2002) Markers of endothelial damage in organ dysfunction and sepsis. Crit Care Med 30:S302–S312

36. Duranteau J, Sitbon P, Teboul JL et al (1999) Effects of epinephrine, norepinephrine or the combination of norepinephrine and dobutamine on gastric mucosa in septic shock. Crit Care Med 27:893–900

37. Li H, Forstermann U (2000) Nitric oxide in the pathogenesis of vascular disease. J Pathol 190:244–254

38. Petros A, Lamb G, Leone A et al (1994) Effects of a nitric oxide synthase inhibitor in humans with septic shock. Cardiovasc Res 28:34–39

39. Baeuerle P, Henkel T (1994) Function and activation of NF-kB in the immune system. Annu Rev Immunol 12:141–179

40. Christman JW, Lancaster LH, Blackwell TS (1998) Nuclear factor kappa B:a pivotal role in the systemic inflammatory response syndrome and new target for therapy. Intensive Care med 24:1131–1138

41. Senden NH, Jeunhomme TM, Heemskerk JW et al (1998) Factor Xa induces cytokine production and expression of adhesion molecules by human umbilical vein endothelial cells. J Immunol 161:4318–4324

42. Creasey AA, Chang AC, Feigen L et al (1993) Tissue factor pathway inhibitor reduces mortality from Escherichia coli septic shock. J Clin Invest 91:2850–2856

43. Asakura H, Ontachi Y, Mizutani T et al (2001) An enhanced fibrinolysis prevents the development of multiple organ failure in disseminated intravascular coagulation in spite of much activation of blood coagulation. Crit Care Med 29:1164–1168

44. Parry GC, Mackman N (1995) Transcriptional regulation of tissue factor expression in human endothelial cells. Arterioscler Thromb Vasc Biol 15:612–621

45. Levi M, ten Cate H, Bauer KA et al (1994) Inhibition of endotoxin induced activation of coagulation and fibrinolysis by pentoxifylline or by a monoclonal anti-tissue factor antibody in chimpazees. J Clin Invest 93:114–120

46. Conway EM, Rosenberg RD (1988) Tumor necrosis factor suppresses transcription of the thrombomodulin gene in endothelial cells. Mol Cell Biol 8:5588–5592
47. Rosenberg RD, Aird WC (1999) Vascular bed specific hemostasis and hypercoagulable states. N Engl J Med 340:1555–1564
48. Sakata Y, Loskutoff DJ, Gladson CL et al (1986) Mechanism of protein C dependent clot lysis: Role of plasminogen activator inhibitor. Blood 68:1218–1223
49. Murakami K, Okajima K, Uchiba M et al (1996) Activated protein C attenuates endotoxin-induced pulmonary vascular injury by inhibiting activated leukocytes in rats. Blood 87(2):642–647
50. Taylor FB Jr, Chang A, Esmon CT et al (1987) Protein C prevents the coagulopathies and lethal effects of E. coli infusion in the baboon. J Clin Invest 79:918–925
51. Jimenez MF, Marshall J, International Sepsis Forum (2001) Source control in the management of sepsis. Intensive Care Med 27:S49–S62
52. Hanon FX, Monnet DL, Sorensen TL et al (2002) Survival of patients with bacteraemia in relation to initial empirical antimicrobial treatment. Scand J Infect Dis 34:520–528
53. Byl B, Clevenbergh P, Jacobs F et al (1999) Impact of infectious diseases specialists and microbiological data on the appropriateness of antimicrobial therapy of bacteremia. Clin Infect Dis 29:60–66
54. Bochud PY, Glauser MP, Calandra T (2001) Antibiotics in sepsis. Intensive Care Med 27:S33–S48
55. Vincent JL, Jacobs F (2003) Infection in critically ill patients: clinical impact and management. Curr Opin Infect Dis 16:309–313
56. Vincent JL (2002) Sepsis definitions. Lancet Infect Dis 2:135
57. Levy MM, Fink MP, Marshall JC et al. SCCM/ESICM/ACP/ATS/SIS. International Sepsis Definitions Conference. Crit Care Med 2003 31:1250–1256
58. Appoloni O, Dupont E, Andrien M et al (2001) Association of TNF2, a TNF-a promoter gene polymorfism, with plasma TNF a levels and mortality in septic shock. Am J Med 110:486–488
59. Vincent JL, Moreno R, Takala J et al (1996) The SOFA (sepsis related organ failure assessment) score to descrive organ/dysfunction failure. Intensive Care Med 1996:22:707–710
60. Vincent JL, de Mendonca A, Cantraine F et al (1998) Use of the SOFA score to assess the incidence of organ/dysfunction/failure in intensive care units: results of a multicentre, prospective study. Crit Care Med; 26:1793–1800
61. Lundberg JS, Perl TM, Wiblin T et al (1998) Septic shock: an analysis of outcomes for patients with onset on hospital wards versus intensive care units. Crit care med 26:1020–1024
62. Rivers EP, Nguyen HB, Amponsah D (2003) Sepsis: A landscape from the emergency department to the intensive care unit. Crit Care Med 31:968–969
63. Tugrul S, Esen F, Celebi S et al (2002) Reliability of procalcitonin as a severity marker in critically ill patients with inflammatorry response. Anaesth Intensive Care 30:747–754
64. Weil MH, Nakagawa Y, Tang W et al (1999) Sublingual capnometry: a new non-invasive measurement for diagnosis and quantification of severity of circulatory shock. Crit Care Med 27:1225–1229
65. Van den Berghe G, Wouters P, Weekers F et al (2001) Intensive insulin therapy in critically ill. N Engl J Med 345:1359–1367
66. Bochud PY, Glauser MP, Calandra T; International Sepsis Forum (2001) Antibiotics in sepsis: Intensive Care Med 27:S33–S48

67. Fish DN (2002) Optimal antimicrobial therapy for sepsis. Am J Health Syst Pharm 59:S13–S19
68. Vincent JL (2001) Hemodynamic support in septic shock. Intensive Care Med 27: S80–S92
69. Choi PT, Yip G, Quinonez LG et al. Crystalloids vs colloids in fluid resuscitation: A systematic review. Crit Care Med 1999 27:200–210
70. Cook D, Guyatt G (2001) Colloid use for fluid resuscitation: evidence and spin. Ann Intern Med 135:205–208
71. Schierhout G, Roberts I (1998) Fluid resuscitation with colloid or crystalloid solutions in critically ill patients: a systematic review of randomised trials. BMJ 316:961–964
72. Gregory JS, Bonfiglio MF, Dasta JF et al (1991) Experience with phenilephrine as a component of the pharmacologic support of septic shock. Crit Care Med 19:1395–1400
73. Hanneman L, Reinhart K, Grenzer O et al (1995) Comparison of dopamine to dobutamine and norepineprine for oxygen delivery and uptake in septic shock. Crit Care Med 23:1926–1970
74. Jindal N, Hollenberg SM, Dellinger RP (2000) Pharmacologic issues in the management of septic shock. Crit Care Clin 16:233–249
75. Levy B, Bollaert PE, Carpentier C et al (1997) Comparison of norepinephrine for hemodynamics, lactete metabolism, and gastric tonometric variables in septic shock: A prospective, randomized study. Intensive Care Med 23:282–287
76. Dhainaut JF, Yan SB, Cariou A et al (2002) Soluble thrombomodulin, plasma-derived unactivated protein C, and recombinant human activated protein C in sepsis. Crit Care Med 30:S318–S324
77. Bone RC, Fisher CJ, Clemmer TP et al (1987) A controlled clinical trial of high dose methylprednisolone in the treatment of severe sepsis and septic shock. N Engl J Med 317:653–658
78. Krueger WA, Lenhart FP, Neeser G et al (2002) Influence of combined intravenous and topical antibiotic prophylaxis on the incidence of infections, organ dysfunctions, and mortality in critically ill surgical patients: a prospective, stratified, randomized, double-blind, placebo-controlled clinical trial. Am J Respir Crit Care Med 166:1029–1037
79. De Jonge E, Schultz M, Spanjaard L et al (2003) Effects of selective decontamination of the digestive tract on mortality and acquisition of resistant bacteria in intensive care: a randomised controlled trial. Lancet 363:1011–1016
80. Anonymous (2000) Ventilation with lower tidal volumes as compared with traditional tidal volume for acute lung injury and the acute respiratory distress syndrome. The Acute Respiratory Distress Syndrome Network. N Engl J Med 342:1301–1308
81. Liberati A, D'Amico R, Pifferi S et al (2004) Antibiotic prophylaxis to reduce respiratory tract infections and mortality in adults receiving intensive care. Cochrane Database Syst Rev 4:CD000022
82. van Saene HK, Petros AJ, Ramsay G et al (2003) All great truths are iconoclastic: selective decontamination of the digestive tract moves from heresy to level 1 truth. Intensive Care Med 29:677–690
83. Viviani M, Silvestri L, van Saene HK, Gullo A (2005) Surviving Sepsis Campaign Guidelines: selective decontamination of the digestive tract still neglected. Crit Care Med 33:462–463
84. Cronin L, Cook DJ, Carlet J et al (1995) Corticosteroid treatment for sepsis: a critical appraisal and meta-analysis of the literature. Crit Care Med 23:1430–1439

85. Annane D, Sibille V, Troche G et al (2000) A 3-level prognostic classification in septic shock based on cortisol response to corticotropin. JAMA 283:1038–1045
86. Annane D, Sibille V, Charpentier C et al (2002) Effect of treatment with low doses of hydrocortisone and fludrocortisone on mortality in patients with septic shock. JAMA 288:862–871
87. Chen JY (1996) Intravenous immunoglobulin in the treatment of full term and premature new-born with sepsis. J Formos Med Asoc 24:733–742
88. Schedel I, Dreikh H (1991) Treatment of gram-negative septic shock with an immunoglobulin preparation: a prospective randomized clinical trial. Clin Care Med 10:1104–1113
89. Garbett ND, Munro CS, Cole Pj (1989) Opsonic activity of a new intravenous immunoglobulin preparation: pentaglobin compared with sandoglobulin. Clin Experimental Immunol 76:3–12
90. McCallion K, Harkin DW, Gardiner KR (2004) Role of adenosine in immunomodulation: review of the literature. Crit Care Med 32:273–277
91. Moser GH, Schareder J, Deessen A (1989) Turnover of adenosine in plasma of human and dog blood. Am J Physiol 256:C799–C806
92. Fredholm BB (1997) Purines and neutrophil leukocytes. Gen Pharmacol 28:345–350
93. Beral Al, Cerra FB (1994) Multiple organ failure syndrome in the 1990s. Systemic inflammatory response and organ dysfunction. JAMA 271:226–233
94. Cronstein BN, Levin RI, Belanoff J et al (1986) Adenosine: an endogenous inhibitor of neutrophil-mediated injury to endothelial cells. J Clin Invest 78:760–770
95. Bouma MG, van den Wildenberg FA, Buurman WA (1997) The anti-inflammatory potential of adenosine in ischaemia-reperfusion injury:established and putative beneficial actions of a retaliatory metabolite. Shock 8:313–320
96. Thiel M, Holzer K, Kreimeier U (1997) Effects of adenosine on the functions of circulating polymorphonuclear leukocytes during hyperdynamic endotoxemia. Infect Immun 65:2136–2144
97. Belardinelli L, Linden J, Berne RM (1989) The cardiac effects of adenosine. Prog Cardiovasc Dis 32:73–97
98. Hunt T, Hussain Z (1994) Can wound healing be a paradigm for tissue repair? Med Sci Sports Exerc 26:755–758
99. Ayala A, Lomas J (2003) Pathological aspects of apoptosis in severe sepsis and shock? Int J Biochem Cell Biol 35:7–15
100. Lin LH, Hopf WH (2003) Paradigm of the injury-repair continuum during critical illness. Critical Care Med 31:S493–S495
101. Cobb J, Hotchkiss R, Karl IE et al (1996) Mechanisms of cells injury and death. Br J Anaesth 77:3–10
102. Mahidhara R, Billiar T (2000) Apoptosis in sepsis. Crit Care Med 28:N105–N113
103. Papathanassoglou E, Moynihan J, Ackerman MH (2000) Does programmed cell death (apoptosis) play a role in the development of multiple organ dysfunction in critically ill patients? A review and a theoretical framework. Crit Care Med 28:537–549
104. Abraham JA, Whang JL, Tumolo A et al (1986) Human basic fibroblast growth factor: Nucleotide sequence and genomic organization. EMBO J 5:2523–2528
105. Christians E, Yan L, Benjamin IJ (2002) Heat shock factor 1 and heat shock proteins: critical partners in protection against acute cell injury. Crit Care Med 30:S43–S50
106. Kress HG (2001) The doctor's dilemma: the assessment of successful adjunctive immunotherapy in critically ill patients. In: Faist E (ed) Immunological Screening and Immunotherapy in Critically Ill Patients with Abdominal Infections. Springer, Milan, pp 139–156

107. Finch RG (1998) Design of clinical trials in sepsis: problem and pitfalls. J Antimicrob Chemother 42:A95–A102

108. Levy M, Fink MP, Marshall JC et al (2001) SCCM/ESICM/ATS/SIS International Sepsis Definitions Conference. Crit Care Med 31:1250–1256

109. GascheY, Pittet D, Suter PM (1995) Outcome and prognostic factors in bactaeremic sepsis. In: Sibbald WJ, Vincent JL (eds) Clinical trials for the treatment of sepsis. Berlin, Springer-Verlag, p 35

110. Knaus WA, Draper EA, Wagner DP et al (1985) APACHE II: a severity of disease classification system. Crit Care Med 13:818–829

111. Knaus WA, Wagner DP, Harrell FE (1995) What determines prognosis in sepsis? In: Sibbald WJ, Vincent JL (eds) Clinical trials for the treatment of sepsis. Berlin, Springer-Verlag, p 122

112. Graf J, Doig GS, Cook DJ (2002) Randomized, controlled clinical trials in sepsis:Has methodological quality improved over time? Crit Care Med 30:461–472

113. Vincent JL (1995) The 'at risk' patient population. In: Clinical trials for the treatment of sepsis. In: Sibbald WJ, Vincent JL (eds) Clinical trials for the treatment of sepsis. Berlin, Springer-Verlag, p 13

114. Sibbald WJ, Vincent JL (1995) Round table conference on clinical trials for the treatment of sepsis. Crit Care Med 23:394–399

115. Marshall JC (1995) Multiple organ dysfunction syndrome (MODS). In: Sibbald WJ, Vincent JL (eds) Clinical trials for the treatment of sepsis. Berlin, Springer-Verlag

116. Dellinger RP, Carlet JM, Masur H (2004) Surviving sepsis campaign guidelines for management of severe sepsis and septic shock. Crit Care Med 32:858–873

117. Rice TW, Bernard GR (2005) Therapeutic intervention and target for sepsis. Annu Rev Med 56:225–248

How to Evaluate Performance of Adult Intensive Care Units: A 30Year Experience

J.R. Le Gall, E. Azoulay

Introduction

The performance of an Intensive Care unit (ICU) has different aspects. For many years, the performance was synonymous with the standard mortality ratio (SMR). But nowadays, other aspects of performance are considered: from the patients, families, nurses, doctors and provider's points of view. Several studies, on the other hand, have demonstrated the relationship between organisation and performance.

The Oldest Studies of ICU Performance

Two studies have been published, one in 1976, by a French group proposing a way to evaluate the prognosis of ICU patients [1], the other in 1982, comparing the hospital mortality of US and French ICUs for the first time [2].

In 1976, Rapin et al. [1] published 'Les chances de survie des malades hospitalisés dans un service de réanimation' in French (The chances of survival of patients hospitalised in a resuscitation service). In order to define criteria for prognosis for patients hospitalised in intensive care units, 2105 cases of patients treated for an acute life-threatening illness were reviewed over four years. According to severity initial illness, three groups were defined: firstly, initial illnesses, presumably reversible (55.3%); secondly, several initial illness, presumably reversible (27.7%); thirdly, one or several initial illnesses, with at least one of them presumably irreversible (17 %). Total mortality was 31.3%, significantly lower in women than in men. Concerning the groups, mortality was 8.7% in the first, 42,7% in the second ($p < 0.0001$), and 83% in the third ($p < 0.0001$). In any group, prognosis was influenced by the type of initial disease (respiratory, circulatory, renal or metabolic, septic, neurological and hepato-digestive failure). In groups I and II, mortality was greater when high risk factors exist, and increased with age, but remained below 50%. In group III, mortality was the same with or without high risk factors, was not influenced by age, and was always near 90%. Over the 4 years, mortality significantly lessened in group II, from 57% to 29%. It was concluded that treatment in an intensive care unit for life-threatening visceral acute failure has a poor result when this later is related to chronic or presumably non-reversible disorder. In other cases, high risk factors – particularly old age – revealed no contra indication to treatment in intensive care units.

In 1982, Knaus et al. [2] published the first international comparison of hospital mortality rates for ICU patients in USA and France. For the first time, they used a severity score to describe the patients. They showed that the hospital mortality increased from 5% to 75% according to severity. On the other hand, they did not find any statistical difference in adjusted mortality rates between USA and France.

The Standard Mortality Ratio (SMR)

The SMR is the comparison between the probability of hospital mortality (P) and the observed hospital mortality (O). The probability of mortality is estimated by a model using a severity score [3, 4]. This approach is valid only when used with models characterised by excellent calibration and discrimination [5]. The recent scores are objective, built from logistic regression.

In their order of publication, these are the APACHE III [6], the SAPS II [7] and the MPM II [8].We will take SAPS II as our example.

SAPS II

Le Gall et al. published a New Simplified Acute Physiology Score (SAPS II) in 1993 [7] based on a European North American Multicenter Study. They compared the SMR of the participating countries. All of them had a SMR close to 1, which was as expected, since they participated in the development of SAPS II. What was more striking was the difference in hospital mortality rates according to the countries. Two groups of countries were observed. In the first group (France, Italy, Spain and UK), the hospital mortality rate was around 30%. In the second group (Austria Belgium, Finland, Germany, Netherlands, Switzerland, USA and Canada) the hospital mortality ratio rate was close to 20%. Did that mean that the first group was less performing than the second one? Not at all, since the SMR was 1 for every country. It is probable that the patients of the second group were less severe. The ICUs in these countries could treat patients which in other countries are admitted to the recovery room.

Obsolescence of the Probability Models

During the following years, many studies applied to different populations, presented a calibration of the models that was poor. Another observation was that the SMR was decreasing over the years. Considering for instance the SMR according to the SAPS II model, Glance et al. [9] showed that for 24 ICUs studied, the SMR was always lower than 1 (from 0.406 to 0.773). What could be the explanation? We have only hypotheses: obsolescence of the models, change in the case mix, different selection criteria for admission.

Nevertheless, it was fundamental that the statistical qualities of the models be improved, or even new models proposed.

Improvement of the Probability Models

Several attempts have been published in order to improve the probability model.

Customisation

Customisation of the models is changing the equation of probability without altering the severity score. This method is simple, and has been proposed either for specific applications or for a country. Le Gall and Lemeshow have proposed to customise the SAPS II and the MPM II for early septic patients [12]. Moreno [13] and Metnitz [14] have published customised models.

Expanded Models

Knaus et al. [10] proposed an expanded model for septic patients, adding acidosis, cirrhosis and other variables to the APACHE II score.

Le Gall et al. [11] proposed an expanded SAPS II adapted to the French population. The added variables were collected on the first ICU day. Age and sex were entered, as well as the number of hospital days before ICU admission, the patient's location before ICU admission, the clinical category (medical or surgical). No diagnosis was included, apart from medical drug overdose. This for three reasons: the SMR of these patients was 0.2 using the original SAPS II model; the percentage of this diagnosis varied from 0 to 40% according to the ICUs; this diagnosis is simple, obvious, and easy to collect on the first ICU day.

Repetitive Scoring

Some researchers have outlined the fact that the first ICU days were determining in outcome, and particularly the first three days.

Larche et al. [15] observed the evolution of the Logistic Organ

Dysfunction (LOD) model [16] during the first three ICU days in cancer patients. They showed that the difference between the LOD 3 and the LOD 1 was determinant for the prognosis.

Timsit et al. [17] proposed a score based on SAPS II and LOD collected during the first three ICU days. They called this composite score the TRIOS and showed an excellent calibration.

Unpublished Scores

The SAPS III has been developed from a worldwide database of 19 577 patients. The score itself comprises three parts: the chronic variables, the acute variables including the sepsis and its characteristics, and the physiology. The probability of ICU and hospital death is given by adding diagnoses to the model. The evaluation of ICU performance is adapted to each ICU according to its case-mix. The APACHE IV uses the ICU day-one information, from a specific US database of 13 618 consecutive admissions. It is very similar to the APACHE III, but new variables are added and different statistical modelling used.

Other Aspects of Performance

The Patient's Points of View

The patient's points of view are obviously different for dying and surviving patients.

For dying patients, many studies have been published about the management of death in ICU. A book edited by Curtis and Rubenfeld [17], entitled 'Managing death in the Intensive Care Unit, the transition from cure to comfort' has been recently published.

For surviving patients, what is important is the quality of life. Among the numerous papers devoted to this subject, we may quote the article from Herridge et al. [18]. Looking at the one year outcomes of ARDS survivors, they found that 40 patients out of 82 one-year survivors (49%) had returned to work. More, among these 40 patients, 31 (78%) returned to their original work. Considering, on the other hand, the ability to exercise and the health-related quality of life, they found that one year after ICU discharge, 89% of survivors had a normal physical functioning, and 88% a normal social functioning.

The Families' Points of View

Many studies have been published regarding the families' outcome. Let us quote a study by Azoulay et al. [19] about the family members' desire to share in the decision-making process. Poor comprehension was noted in 35% of family members. Among intensive care unit staff members, 91% of physicians and 83% of non-physicians believed that participation in decision-making should be offered to families; however, only 39% had actually involved family members in decisions. A desire to share in decision-making was expressed by only 47% of family members. Only 15% of family members actually shared in decision-making. Effectiveness of information influenced this desire.

The Burn Out Syndrome

Both nurses and doctors may suffer from burn out syndrome, the exhaustion due to physical and psychological burdens. One study by Embriaco et al. [20], showed that 46.5% of 959 intensive care staff it interviewed on one day had a high degree of burn out. The high risk factors of burn out were shown to be: being female, having too many duties, too few holidays and conflicts between doctors or with nurses.

Relationship Between Management and Performance

Good management makes for good performance. The first study published about this relationship was the Shortell et al. study [21]. Based on data collected from 17 440 patients across 42 ICUs, the study examines the factors associated with risk-adjusted mortality, risk-adjusted average length of stay, nurse turnover, evaluated technical quality of care, and evaluated ability to meet family member needs. Using the APACHE III methodology for risk-adjustment, findings reveal that: 1) technological availability is significantly associated with lower risk-adjusted mortality (beta = 0.42); 2) diagnostic diversity is significantly associated with greater risk-adjusted mortality (beta = 0.43); and 3) care-giver interaction comprising the culture, leadership, co-ordination, communication, and conflict management abilities of the unit is significantly associated with lower risk-adjusted length of stay (beta = 0.34), lower nurse turnover (beta = 0.36), higher evaluated technical quality of care (beta = 0.81), and greater evaluated ability to meet family member needs (beta = 0.74). Furthermore, units with greater technological availability are significantly more likely to be associated with hospitals that are more profitable, involved in teaching activities, and have unit leaders actively participating in hospital wide quality improvement activities.

A French study by Azoulay et al. [22] on 920 families showed the positive factors influencing the satisfaction of patients' families. These are: family members of French descent, patient to nurse ratio ≤ 3, information provided by junior physicians and family helped by their usual doctor. On the other side, the negative factors were: family feeling they received contradictory information, family not knowing the specific role of each care-giver, desired/allowed time ratio.

Conclusions

To evaluate an ICU performance the SMR is necessary (but not sufficient). The SMR must be calculated using customised or expanded scores. The first three ICU days are fundamental for the outcome.

The performance must take into account the patients, families and personal points of view.

We must stress that good management makes for a high-performing unit.

References

1. Rapin M, Gomez Duque A, Le Gall JR et al (1976) Les chances de survie des malades hospitalisés dans un service de réanimation. Nouv Presse Med 6:1245–1248
2. Knaus WA, Le Gall JR, Wagner DP et al (1982) A comparison of intensive care in the USA and France. Lancet 2:642–646
3. Le Gall JR, Loirat P (1995) Can we evaluate the performance of an Intensive Care Unit? Curr Opin Crit Care 1:219–220
4. Ridley S (1998) Severity of illness scoring systems and performance appraisal. Anaesthesia 12:1185–1194
5. Lemeshow S, Le Gall JR (1994) Modeling the severity of illness of ICU patients. A system update JAMA 272:1049–1055
6. Knaus WA, Drape EA, Wagner DP et al (1985) APACHE II: a severity of disease classification system. Crit Care Med 13:819–829
7. Le Gall JR, Lemeshow S, Saulnier F (1993) A new Simplified Acute Physiologic Score (SAPS II) based on an European/North American multicenter study. JAMA 270:2957–2963
8. Lemeshow S, Teres D, Klar J et al (1993) Mortality Probability Models (MPH II) based on an international cohort of intensive care unit patients. JAMA 270:2478–2486
9. Glance LG, Osler TM, Dick A (2002) Rating the quality of Intensive Care Units: Is it a function of the ICU scoring system? Crit Care Med 30(9):1976–1982
10. Knaus WA, Harrel FE, Fischer CJ H Jr et al (1993) The clinical evaluation of new drugs for sepsis: a prospective study design based on survival analysis. JAMA 270:1233–1240
11. Le Gall JR, Neumann A, Hemery F et al (2005) Expanding the SAPS II Improves Mortality Prediction. Reanimation, 14(suppl 1):
12. Le Gall JR, Lemeshow S, Leleu G et al (1995) Customized probability models for early severe sepsis in adult intensive care patients. JAMA 273:644–650
13. Moreno R, Apolone G (1997) Impact of different customization strategies in the performance of a general severity score. Crit Care Med 25:2001–2008

14. Metnitz P, Lang T, Vesely H et al (2000) Ratios of observed to expected mortality are affected by difference in case mix and quality of care. Int Care Med 26:1466–1472

15. Larche J, Azoulay E, Fieux F et al (2003) Improved survival of critically ill cancer patients with septic shock. Int Care Med 29:1688–1697

16. Le Gall JR, Klar J, Lemeshow S et al (1996) The Logistic Organ Dysfunction system. A new way to assess organ dysfunction in the intensive care unit. ICU Scoring Group. JAMA 276(10):802–810

17. Curtis JR, Rubenfeld GD (eds) (2001) Managing death in the ICU: the transition from cure to comfort. Oxford, Oxford University Press

18. Herridge MS, Cheung AM, Tansey CM et al (2003) One-year outcomes in survivors of the acute respiratory distress syndrome. N Engl J Med 348(8):683–693

19 Azoulay E, Pochard F, Chevret S et al (2004) Half the family members of intensive care unit patients do not want to share in the decision making process: A study in 78 French Intensive care units. Crit Care Med 32:1832–1838

20. Embriaco N, Barrau K, Azoulay E et al (2005) Prévalence et facteurs de risque du burn out chez les réanimateurs français. Reanimation 14(suppl 1) SOE 27

21. Shortell SR, Zimmerman JE, Gillies RR et al (1994) The performance of Intensive Care Unit: does good management make a difference? Med Care 32:508–525

22. Azoulay E, Pochard F, Chevret S et al (2001) Meeting the needs of Intensive care unit patient families – a multicenter study. Am J Resp Crit Care Med 163:135–139

Research Ethics in Critical Care Medicine

P.D. Lumb

Research in critical care medicine is founded on the trust of our patients and their families. In order to understand the integrity of this mutually responsible relationship, it is important to review the foundations upon which it is built. Two core questions define our understanding of the importance between the patient's expectations and our inherent clinical responsibilities. It is equally important to recognise that much of what has become today's accepted critical care practice derives from uncontrolled clinical experimentation that each of us perform in the context of providing optimal patient care. Therefore it is important to understand the founding principles of the ethical considerations of patient care and research in the intensive care unit (ICU): Where do the principles come from and what do we learn from their application?

Stated simply, there are four concepts: beneficence, non-maleficence, respect for persons, and justice. It is more important, however, to understand what they mean and how they apply to patient care in the current environment in which accountability, transparency, and increasingly informed consumers are creating an environment that is much different from the paternalistic climate in which medicine was practiced for centuries. Indeed, the present state provides for increased opportunity as outcomes-based therapeutic interventions become standard practice. *Primum non nocere*, first do no harm; a simple sounding phrase, but it is the core of an interesting argument between research and routine in practice. Ethical principles are important because they are the foundation of all legitimate research with, and the care of, human beings. Equally, they inspire and support society's confidence in research concepts and support biomedical research autonomy while providing useful tools that aid in the design, approval, and adjudication of research protocols. Finally, they serve as a set of specific rules and procedures that enforce humanity and humility.

Three interesting viewpoints are shown in the writings of individuals whose reputations stand for ethical, humane treatment. Moses Maimonides (1135-1204) believed that patients were ends in themselves and should not be used as a 'means of learning new truths', while Roger Bacon (1214-1294) stated that 'the body demands that no error be made in operating upon it and so experience is so difficult in medicine'. It is interesting to note the significant difference in the experience of Walter Reed, whose 'Yellow Fever contract' indicated that his 'volunteers' preferred to intentionally risk contracting yellow fever because it was implied that by so doing they would receive the 'greatest care and most skillful medical service'. As an added incentive to volunteer, those soldiers who agreed to be exposed to yellow fever were promised payment in gold, a significant inducement at the time. It appears that Reed felt the disease to be so endemic in the region, and that its isolation and treatment were so important, that this type of experimentation was warranted. Today's institutional review boards (IRB) and practicing physicians may feel differently.

The first signs of research controls relevant today appear in a 1900 series of Prussian prohibitions that included the following concepts: the competency of the experimental subject must be confirmed; full disclosure of experimental risk must be provided to the subject and/or surrogate; and informed consent must be obtained. At Nuremberg, additional safeguards were introduced that included: the concept of 'voluntary' consent; that the results of the experiment were anticipated to be fruitful and for the good of society; and that the subject should be at liberty to discontinue the experiment at any time. It is interesting to note that after World War II and the introduction of the Nuremberg Code, in which Principles 1 and 9 restate the importance of voluntary consent and the ability to discontinue the experiment respectively, and despite the recognised abuses to individuals during internment, many physicians viewed the problem as primarily belonging to a particular place and time, i.e. Nazi Germany, and was not seen as relevant to their practice. This belief was shattered by publications in the United States that revealed the extent to which experimental subjects required protection and that a definition of subject protection that included incarcerated individuals had to be established. Also, the influence of experimental design and appropriate application of statistical methods leading to justifiable conclusions became a troublesome topic. Specifically, two studies – the 1966 New England Journal of Medicine Beecher Study indicating that analysis and therefore conclusions in large numbers of publications were flawed and the 1972 exposure of the results of the Tuskegee syphilis study in which US federal inmates were denied treatment in order to allow the disease to progress naturally – indicated that even under the 'best' circumstances, experimentation had to be controlled.

The breach of medical and ethical trust leading to the requirement for and consequences of the Nuremberg declarations occurred because the intent of experimentation was not to investigate outcomes of the scientific application of clinical protocols designed to promote the healing process. Rather, the investigation concluded that blatant experiments on humans that was in no way motivated by a therapeutic premise had been performed. It is recognised that the consequences of participation in a controlled clinical trial may be, and in some cases tragically, unexpected. Nonetheless, there must be the underlying expectation and principle that therapeutic benefit underpins the therapeutic regimen and that outcome will be closely watched and appropriate interventions to terminate unnecessary studies made if interim data analysis warrants such action.

The above statements underscore the importance of respect for persons that is one of the cardinal beliefs in the management of medical research endeavours. Respect for persons incorporates the following two convictions: those individuals should be treated as autonomous agents and that persons with decreased autonomy are entitled to protection. Despite the fact that these principles have been mentioned above, it is the following actions that must be implemented. There is an inherent requirement for all medical investigators to recognise an individual patient's autonomy and that, especially in critical care practice, individuals with diminished autonomy must be provided protection. It is largely in this area that current critical care research is both hampered and aided.

The concept of beneficence is an easy one to understand and simply stated indicates that physicians should do no harm to their patients, and should always attempt to maximise possible benefits while minimising possible harms of therapeutic intervention. The obligations of beneficence affect individual investigators, the institutions in which they work, research sponsoring organisations, and society at large because they underpin the framework of human investigation. Development of IRB's and pharmaceutical watchdog panels have developed in the past few years, yet today's headlines and National Public Radio broadcasts still retain the ability to shock. Recent allegations that Merck attempted to hide early reports of Vioxx's cardiac danger are now being defended; yet, superficial arguments have already lost the public's trust in the company and make ongoing enrollment in current clinical investigations increasingly difficult. In the case of particular projects, investigators and their institutions are obliged to give forethought to the maximisation of benefits and the reduction of risk that might occur from the research investigation.

Despite numerous false steps, principles alluded to in the preceding discussion have become more formally adopted in a number of well established rules. Namely, respect for a person is easily recognised as the well-established requirement to obtain informed consent from any study participant, and the concept of beneficence requires that odds ratios and risk minimisation are taken into account when designing experimental protocols. Statistical avenues must be available that will indicate if and when studies need to be terminated, either because the results are unexpectedly good and it would be unfair to withhold therapy from non-participants, or the converse. Justice is easily identified as the common practice to include multiple ethnic and cultural populations in any trial; certainly, no racial selection bias is acceptable, especially if there is a presupposition of increased benefit to be derived from study participation.

There is an increased public awareness that in order to advance medical therapeutics and interventions human experimentation is required. Therefore, a new tension is apparent in the ethical undertaking of new clinical interventions and therapeutic trials. Redefinition of the situation in which the ethics codified at Nuremberg and in prior thought and practice (Maimonides, Bacon) equaled subject protection to the current requirement of medical innovation in which ethical principles must provide access to human subjects for medical therapeutic trials is necessary. This is a difficult paradox because all investigators understand that while research can never be considered therapy, nonetheless research entry may lead to therapeutic benefit. Indeed, no clinician would knowingly enter patients into trials in which the likelihood of a neutral or improved outcome was clearly reduced. Therefore, despite the requirement for improved clinical studies in increasingly acute situations in which subject autonomy is likely reduced, the medical profession is coming under increased scrutiny and suspicion because of highly profiled failures in the ethical codes in which we all have great confidence and trust. To a certain extent, increased complexity in the science of medicine and the reduction of its art have helped create an environment that is more error prone and likely to cause harm from a myriad of systems related problems that have little to do with medical ethics or therapeutic experimentation. Despite the obvious differences in these areas, the lines between them are indistinctly drawn and the propensity to confuse the boundaries is commonplace.

In clinical practice, the extensions of some of the previously discussed principles have become well-recognised guidelines, policies, or procedures. For example, recent institution of the Healthcare Information Portability and Privacy Act (HIPPA) is an example of a perhaps overly rigorous application of the value that each patient is autonomous and that information collected about him is confidential and should be made available to the patient or designee freely. Equally responsive to the concepts of autonomy are the regulations surrounding do not resuscitate (DNR) orders, the concept of advanced health care directives and the discussions surrounding the withdrawal of life support. Indeed recent events in the United States and Italy underscore the differing manner in which quality of life and autonomy have been interpreted, politicised, and ultimately confused for lay public and medical investigation advocate alike.

Additional concerns and complicating factors are in evidence throughout medical practice. Increasingly the use of advanced technology and therapeutics is confusing the borders between the possible and the ethically and morally practical. Limits on treatment are challenged in public forums, and increasingly sophisticated arguments are invoked to create new ethical challenges to an already complicated environment. From a practical standpoint, overcrowded hospitals and emergency departments are constantly faced with triage decisions that strain the physician-patient relationship and further complicate the concepts of therapeutic justice that demand individuals receive a fair share of the resources committed to medical intervention based on their need. Additional thought leaders have added that resource allocation may also consider an individual's effort, contributions to society, and merit in allocating scarce resources. This is scarcely a popular discussion point in societies that feel that medical care is an entitlement, yet it is a daily reality in world populations where the purchase of anti-malarial drugs is beyond the financial means of many, despite the fact that in western terms it is a trivially small sum. Similar concerns are noted in the distribution of anti-HIV medications in Africa. It will be interesting to note whether or not the recent G-8 Financial Summit decision to forgive debt to a number of African and Latin American countries will alleviate some of these discrepancies. Somehow, it appears unlikely that early investments will flow to the medical infrastructure.

Perhaps one of the more difficult and misunderstood aspects of medical care and research relates to the increasing likelihood that the moral, ethical, religious, and societal beliefs of patient and practitioner may differ. As the world's borders shrink, and travel between nations becomes ubiquitous and ethnic communities become commonplace, often the very institutions that were developed to care for a homogenous patient population are now dealing with an entirely different set of problems and cultural challenges. Interpreters, priests, rabbis, imams, and monks to name a few are essential participants in patient care in our institution. It is scarcely surprising that some of the medical decisions that appear commonplace in a western culture are questioned and rejected in others. Institutions and practitioners must become sensitive to the needs of other and not personally held beliefs. It is for this and many other reasons that a strong understanding of and adherence to ethical principles be communicated to all members of the health-care team.

The new paradigm is that healthcare should be safe and effective, centred on the patient, delivered in a timely and efficient manner, and accountable to the study of outcomes of similar therapies over time, different populations, and institutions. Also, it is anticipated that the rendered care will be equitable and responsible to society. In the 2001 publication, *Crossing the Quality Chasm*, Richardson writes the following recommendations for a code of conduct in health care. He states:

'Care should be based on continuous healing relationships. The health care system should be responsive at all times, and access to care should be provided over the Internet, by telephone, and by other means in addition to face-to-face visits.

Care should be customised based on patient needs and values. The system of care should be designed to meet the most common types of needs, but have the capability to respond to individual patient choices and preferences.

Control should reside with the patient. Patients should be given the necessary information and the opportunity to exercise the degree of control they choose over health-care decisions that affect them.

Knowledge and information should be shared with the patient. Patients should have unfettered access to their own medical information and to clinical knowledge.

Clinical decisions should be evidence-based, that is, patients should receive care based on the best scientific evidence.

The care system should be safe. Patients should not have to worry about injury.

The health system should be more transparent and make information available to patients and their families that allows them to make informed decisions when selecting a health plan, hospital, or clinical practice, or when choosing among alternative treatments.

The health system should anticipate patient needs rather than simply reacting to events.

The health system should not waste resources or patient time.

There should be more cooperation among clinicians to ensure an appropriate exchange of information and coordination of care.' [1]

These comments are reminiscent of the preceding discussion and codify ethical principles into a more readable and interpretable form than previously available. It is also more comprehensive and demands greater societal accountability than the patients' Bill of Rights readily available in most American hospitals.

An earlier Institute of Medicine report published in 1999 is the prequel to the above and was the first public admission that there may be a problem in American Healthcare that was rooted in traditional practice and was either unaware of significant systemic and dangerous practices in many institutions or unwilling to recognise and admit to the failings in order to solve identifiable problems. In part, the report indicates that:

Current scientific publication (results of controlled clinical trials, multi-centre reviews, results of new drug formulations or medical techniques, etc.) should be joined by discussions of ethical and quality-improvement issues seasoned with administrative techniques that target cost effective and socially responsible practice. It must be understood that there is a greater public sophistication and interest in the outcome of individual and population-based therapeutic initiatives. Many patients arrive in the physician's office or anaesthesia pre-screening area armed with the latest 'Googled' information about new therapeutic innovations and elevated expectations regarding the likely outcomes of therapy. Recent public interest in patient safety has become a major concern of healthcare regulators, and the influence of this aspect of patient care coupled with the importance of understanding the ethical basis of medical practice can be seen in the Joint Commission on Accreditation of Healthcare Organizations (JCAHO) 2005 initiative [2] that encompasses the following seven institutional requirements:

1. Improve the accuracy of patient information
2. Improve effectiveness of communication among caregivers
3. Improve safety of using high-alert medications
4. Improve the safety of infusion pumps
5. Reduce risk of health care-acquired infection
6. Accurately and completely reconcile medications across the continuum of care
7. Reduce the risk of patient harm resulting from falls

Further attention to this topic followed an Oprah Winfrey Television program advertised as follows:

'A woman had a hysterectomy and went through chemotherapy – but she never had cancer.

A man woke from surgery – without his penis.

Discover what you need to know before you go to any doctor.'

The program aired at a time when the United States was recovering from a series of highly publicised medical errors that included a mismatched transplant in a well-known and respected institution, and the stories of swapped babies in two Boston hospitals. Undoubtedly errors in management occur; each of us must embrace the technologic and work-environment (cultural) improvements necessary to insure safe, effective and responsible patient care.

In order to understand the relationship between ethical treatment of patients and the attention paid to medical error, it is important to recognise that each of us works within the context of a system that determines the success or failure of our initiatives. The following definitions may be helpful in rationalising the connection:

- Safety: Safety is defined as freedom from accidental injury [3]
- Accident: An accident is an event that involves damage to a defined system that disrupts the ongoing or future output of that system [4]
- Error: Error is defined as the failure of a planned action to be completed as intended (i.e. Error of execution) or the use of a wrong plan to achieve an aim (e.g. Error of planning) [3]
- Active Errors: Active errors occur at the level of the front-line operator, and their effects are felt almost immediately. This is sometimes called the 'sharp end'
- Latent Errors: Latent errors tend to be removed from the direct control of the operator and include things such as poor design, incorrect installation, faulty maintenance, bad management decisions, and poorly structured organisations [3]
- System: A system is a set of interdependent elements interacting to achieve a common aim. The elements may be both human and non-human (equipment, technologies, etc.) [5]
- Human Factors (study): Human factors is defined as the study of the interrelationships between humans, the tools they use, and the environment in which they live and work [6]

It is important to understand the concept of a system because much of what we do and discuss lies within the context of a healthcare system. A system is a whole that cannot be divided into independent parts and its defining function or property derives from the interactions of its parts, not their actions taken separately. Therefore, a system functions as a set of interrelated units that are (theoretically) engaged in joint problem-solving with the express intent to accomplish a unified goal, in this case the safe, effective, and humane care of patients relevant to society. With this understanding, the following questions are relevant and presuppose a greater understanding of Quality Improvement initiatives that are now ubiquitous in medical care.

- Why is it a trap to look for defects?
- Why is it better to do the right thing wrong than to do the wrong thing right?
- Define the difference between cooperative competition and destructive conflict.
- An improvement program must be directed at what you want, not at what you don't want

These questions provide the unifying argument that relates critical care research paradigms to the requirement to understand medical decision making and the underlying importance of the governance and practice systems in which we work and administer patient care. The function of a medical audit is to:

- Improve quality of medical care

- Compare actual with agreed upon standards of practice
- Provide a formal, systematic, and peer reviewed/responsive accounting of rendered care
- Identify and investigate deviations between practice performance and an agreed upon or idealised standard
- Provide criteria measurement for continuous review and improvement

It is only through our participation in these activities that the processes, effectiveness, and outcome of care delivery can be improved. Equally, it can be argued that in order to accomplish the goals of a medical audit, some degree of medical experimentation is required. Whether or not this falls under the auspices of an IRB or a Medical Staff oversight committee remains an interesting question. The answer is important to our practice and our autonomy as physicians. Equally, the following statements reflect our current situation and vulnerability.

'The Sicilians never want to improve for the simple reason they think themselves perfect; their vanity is stronger than their misery.' [7]

'Health care systems fail to provide treatments that are known to work, persist in using treatments that don't work, enforce delays, and tolerate high levels of error.' [8]

Are we in a position that although we understand the necessity for change, we are incapable of initiating the necessary processes through which improvement in the quality and efficacy of the treatments we prescribe can be effected? Experience and history provide a confused answer to this disturbing question. Despite the fact that Semmelweiss was ridiculed for his insistence on hand washing to diminish the incidence of puerperal fever, and despite the fact that today's physicians adhere to the principles of asepsis, it is interesting to note that in multiple surveys of hospital practice, physicians are some of the worst offenders in their lack of routine hand washing between patient contacts and when moving from isolation facilities. It should not come as a surprise that the JCAHO has made 'hand hygiene' an additional accreditation standard and focus of inspector attention during site surveys. It appears that despite a well recognised, outcome credible mechanism to reduce hospital infections and morbidity, we apparently ignore good practice standards while advocating more sophisticated and invasive technologies that are increasingly prone to complications related to poor technique.

However, a slightly different question poses the ethical and research dilemmas that are implied in this discussion. Sonography is a well recognised imaging modality that has multiple medical applications. Many cardiac anaesthesiologists are experienced in the application of trans-oesophageal echocardiography (TEE) and have acquired practice credentials for its use either through certification by examination and/or institutional medical staff credentialing bodies. Indeed, in many centres, routine use of TEE is the norm and residency and fellowship training programs provide basic instruction in its use. However, the use of sonographic imaging techniques for insertion of central venous and arterial catheters and for the performance of nerve blocks is less the standard of care than the advent of a technique that promises to provide greater safety in the performance of these procedures. The practical impact of this statement is not only in the practical, financial cost of providing the equipment, but also in the training time and cost of instructing individuals in its use. Introduction of any new technology or therapeutic intervention requires meticulous attention to the details of its use and demands familiarity with the equipment itself. These are non-controversial statements. The crux of this discussion focuses on the mechanism through which the technology or intervention is introduced into patient care. Despite the fact that a practitioner has placed multiple catheters successfully without sonographic guidance, does the first placement with the device constitute an experiment that requires informed patient consent? Equally, when faced with a clinical assessment of an individual who may have a compromised airway, does the utilisation of a fiberoptic intubation by a less experienced practitioner create a more dangerous patient care situation, despite its support by current custom and publications? The important issues surrounding our daily care are not that clinical decisions can and should not be made. Rather, the underlying principles of research ethics must permeate all aspects of care, rather than just those covered by IRB protocol.

'Physicians today are experiencing frustration as changes in the healthcare delivery system in virtually all industrialised countries threaten the very nature and values of medical professionalism. Medicine's commitment to the patient is being challenged by external forces of change within our societies.' [9]. This statement underscores the importance to understand the stimulus and mechanisms of change present in the medical environments in which we work, and the importance of the ethical principles on which our profession is founded. Equally, the current principles on which we practice and are judged and the challenges we face today are forecast by Hippocrates in the following statements:

'I will apply dietetic measures for the benefit of the sick according to my *ability* and *judgment*; I will keep them from harm and injustice.

I will neither give a deadly drug to anybody who asked for it, nor will I make a suggestion to this effect. In purity and holiness I will guard my life and my art.

What I may see or hear in the course of the treatment or even outside of the treatment on regard to the life of men, which on no account one must be spread abroad, I will keep to myself, holding such things shameful to be spoken about.' [10]

These are some of the reasons why it is important to understand the ethical foundation on which we practice. First, and as discussed previously, ethical considerations have significant impact on decision making in acute care settings. Second, principles derived from the study of medical ethics are needed to respond appropriately in the acute/critical care environment when the situation demands our best and immediate attention. The outcomes of these interventions must be subjected to peer review, and when indicated, changes in practice management must be effected in order to improve the quality, efficacy, and safety of patient care. The goal is to improve quality of care by identifying, analysing, and resolving moral and management questions arising in clinical practice. Ethical principles provide the bridge that enables us to link the practical and the ethereal.

Perhaps the Chinese philosopher Lao-tzu most eloquently expressed the difficulty in linking these concepts in the following statements:

We join spokes together in a wheel,
but it is the centre hole that makes the wagon move.

We shape clay into a pot,
But it is the emptiness inside that holds whatever we want.

We hammer wood for a house,
But it is the inner space that makes it livable.

We work with being,
But non-being is what we use. [11]

References

1. Richardson W (2001) Crossing the Quality Chasm: A New Health System for the 21st Century; Institute of Medicine, Public Briefing, March 1
2. Anonymous (2005) Setting the Standard. The Joint Commission on Accreditation of Healthcare Organizations, p 5, available at http://www.jcaho.org/general+public/patient+safety/setting_the_standard.pdf, last accessed on June 2005
3. Kohn LT, Corrigan JM, Donaldson MS (eds) (1999) To err is human. Building a safer health system. Washington, DC, National Academy Press
4. Perrow C (1984) Normal accidents, New York
5. Reason J (1990) Human error. Cambridge, Cambridge University Press
6. Weinger MB, Pantiskas C, Wiklund M et al (1998) Incorporating human factors into the design of medical devices. JAMA, 280:1484
7. Giuseppe Tomasi di Lampedusa, *The Leopard*

8.   Smith R (2001) Change: both desired and resisted. BMJ :322
9.   ABIM Foundation; American Board of Internal Medicine; ACP-ASIM Foundation. American College of Physicians-American Society of Internal Medicine; European Federation of Internal Medicine (2002) Medical professionalism in the new millennium: a physician charter. Ann Intern Med 136:243-246
10. Ludwig Edelstein (ed) (1943) The Hippocratic Oath. Text, Translation, and Interpretation by Ludwig Edelstein. Johns Hopkins Press, Baltimore
11. Lao-tzu. Tao Te Ching, 4th Century BC

Scoring Systems and Outcome

R. Moreno, P. Metnitz

Introduction

The evaluation of severity of illness in the critically ill patient is made through the use of severity scores and prognostic models. Severity scores are instruments that aim at stratifying patients based on the severity of illness, assigning to each patient an increasing score as their severity of illness increases. Prognostic models, apart from their ability to stratify patients according to their severity, predict a certain outcome (usually the vital status at hospital discharge) based on a given set of prognostic variables and a certain modeling equation.

The development of these kinds of systems, applicable to heterogeneous groups of critically ill patients, started in the 1980s.

The first general severity of illness score applicable to most critically ill patients was the Acute Physiology and Chronic Health Evaluation (APACHE) [1]. Developed at the George Washington University Medical Centre in 1981 by William Knaus et al., the APACHE system demonstrated the ability to evaluate, in an accurate and reproducible form, the severity of disease in this population [2-4].

Two years later, Jean-Roger Le Gall and co-workers published a simplified version of this model, the Simplified Acute Physiology Score (SAPS) [5]. This model soon became very popular in Europe, especially in France.

Another simplification of the original APACHE system, the APACHE II, was published in 1985 by the same authors of the original model [6]. This system introduced the possibility to predict mortality, needing for this purpose the selection of a major reason for intensive care unit (ICU) admission from a list comprising 50 operative and non-operative diagnoses. Additional contributions for the prediction of prognosis comprise the Mortality Probability Models (MPM) [7], developed by Stanley Lemeshow using logistic regression techniques.

The last developments in this field include the third version of the APACHE system (APACHE III) [8] and the second versions of the SAPS (SAPS II) [9] and MPM (MPM II) [10]. All of them used multiple logistic regression to select and weigh the variables, and are able to compute the probability of hospital mortality for groups of critically ill patients. It has been demonstrated that they perform better than their old counterparts [11, 12], and they represent nowadays the state-of-the-art in this field. However, a new generation of general outcome prediction models is now being developed, such as the MPM III developed in the IMPACT database in the United States of America (USA) [13]. In addition there are new models based on computerised analysis by hierarchical regression developed by some of the authors of the APACHE systems [14] or the new version of the SAPS model, developed by hierarchical regression in a worldwide database (Rui Moreno, personnel communication, www.saps3.org for more details). Models based on other statistical techniques such as artificial neural networks and genetic algorithms have been proposed but besides academics use they have never been widely used [15, 16].

Given the general character of this chapter, we will not present or discuss instruments developed for particular conditions; for specific issues, the reader should consult specific reviews, such as for paediatrics [17], cardiac surgery [18], trauma [19-21] or risk of sepsis [22].

Also, due to the general structure of this chapter, we will not revise scores designed for the quantification and description of multiple organ dysfunction failure [23-25] or mixed systems [26]. The reader can find some guidelines of their use in Moreno et al. [27] and in Bernard [28].

The Existing Models

APACHE II

APACHE II was developed based on data registered between 1979 and 1982 in 13 hospitals of the USA [6]. The choice of variables and their weights was selected by a group of experts, using clinical judgment and physiological relationships as documented in the literature.

The model uses the most deranged value from the first 24 hours in the ICU of 12 physiological variables (scored from 0 to 4 points), age, surgical status (emergency surgery, scheduled surgery or non-operative), and previous health status. A main reason for ICU admission has to be chosen from a list of 50 operative and non-operative diagnoses, in order to transform the APACHE II score into a probability of death (in the hospital). The APACHE II score varies from 0 to 71 points: up to 60 for physiological variables, up to 6 for age and up to 5 for previous health status. This system became the most widely used of the general outcome prediction systems, and today it is still used in a large number of ICUs.

APACHE III

The APACHE III system was developed in 1988-89 based on a sample of critically ill patients from 40 hospitals in the USA [8]. The selection of the participating hospitals was intended to be representative of American hospitals with more than 200 beds. Patients with an ICU length of stay less than 4 hours, age < 16 years or an admission diagnosis of burn injury, acute myocardial infarction or coronary artery bypass surgery, were excluded from the cohort.

The model consists of the Acute Physiology Score (APS), age, and chronic health status. The equation uses the APACHE III score and reference data from the main diagnostic categories, the surgical status, and the location of the patient before ICU admission to estimate the vital status at hospital discharge. The APACHE III scores vary between 0 and 299 points, including up to 252 points for the 18 physiological variables, up to 24 points for age, and up to 23 points for the chronic health status. All the physiological variables are evaluated as the most deranged values from the first 24 hours in the ICU. This strategy was chosen by the authors to minimise the amount of missing data and to increase the explanatory power of the model [8], but eventually there are pitfalls when the model is used to evaluate the performance of the ICU [29].

The computation of the probability of mortality is made using individual logistic regression coefficients for each one of 78 acute diagnosis and 9 locations before ICU admission. APACHE III, however, is marketed as a commercial system and a specific software for the calculation of hospital mortality has thus to be purchased from the developers. This fact severely limited its use, specially outside the USA. Nevertheless, APACHE III has also been applied in other countries such as Brazil [30, 31], Spain [32] and the United Kingdom [33–35].

SAPS II

The SAPS II was described in 1993 by Jean-Roger Le Gall et al. based on the European-North American Study (ENAS) database [9]. It was developed in a large sample of 110 hospitals in Europe and 27 hospitals in North America. Patients < 18 years of age or with a main diagnosis of burns, acute ischaemic heart disease, and cardiac surgery were excluded.

This model includes 17 variables: 12 physiologic variables, age, type of admission (non-operative and emergency/elective surgery) and three chronic diagnoses (AIDS, metastatic cancer and haematological cancer). The SAPS II model uses, as seen previously systems, the most deranged physiologic values registered during the first 24 hours in the ICU. The SAPS II score can vary between 0 and 163 points (up to 116 points for physiological variables, up to 17 points for age and up to 30 points for previous diagnosis).

MPM II

The MPM II was described by Stanley Lemeshow et al. in 1993 [10]. Based on the same database that was used for the development of the SAPS II, with additional data from six ICUs in four American hospitals. Exclusion criteria were the same as those used for the development of the SAPS II model. In the MPM II models, the final result is not expressed as a score, but only as a probability of hospital mortality. The actual version includes models to predict mortality at hospital discharge based on data from admission (MPM II_0) and after the first 24 hours in the ICU (MPM II_{24}). Later, the same authors developed additional models (based on a smaller sample) based on data from 48 hours (MPM II_{48}) and 72 hours after admission to the ICU (MPM II_{72}) [36].

The MPM II_0 model uses 15 variables: age, three physiological variables (coma or deep stupor, heart rate, and systolic blood pressure), three chronic diseases (chronic renal failure, cirrhosis and metastatic cancer), five acute diagnoses (acute renal failure, cardiac arrhythmias, cerebro-vascular incident, gastrointestinal haemorrhage and intracranial mass effect), type of admission (non-operative or emergency surgery), mechanical ventilation and cardiopulmonary resuscitation prior to hospital admission. All these variables are evaluated based on data collected in the first hour before and after ICU admission. An updated version based on the project IMPACT database (USA), has just been published as an abstract [13].

The MPM II_{24} is based on 13 variables: age, six physiological variables (coma or deep stupor, creatinine, documented infection, hypoxaemia, prothrombine time and urinary output), three variables evaluated at ICU admission (cirrhosis, intracranial mass effect, and metastatic cancer), type of admission (non-operative, emergency surgery), mechanical ventilation, and use of vasoactive drugs. The physiological variables are based on the most deranged values during the first 24 hours in the ICU.

The MPM II_{48} and the MPM II_{72} use the same variables as MPM II_{24}, with different weights to compute the probabilities of death and are based on the most deranged values of the preceding 24 hours.

The Application of the Models

All existing models aim to predict an outcome (vital status at hospital discharge) based on a given set of variables: they estimate the outcome of a patient with a certain clinical condition (defined by the registered variables), treated in a hypothetical reference ICU. Several issues, however, need to be taken into account in order to apply one of the above described models in another population:
- Patient selection

- Evaluation and registration of the predictive variables
- Evaluation and registration of the outcome
- Computation of the severity score
- Transformation of the score into a probability of death

Patient Selection

Although named 'general', none of the existing models are applicable to all ICU patients. Patients with burns, admitted with coronary ischaemia (or to rule-out myocardial infarction), young (less than 16 or 18 years of age), in the post-operative of cardiac surgery, or with a very short length of ICU stay where explicitly excluded from their development.

This limitation is especially important when we evaluate specialised ICUs, with a particular case mix, but it can also be important in general ICUs. In many cases, the application of exclusion criteria can involve the analysis of just a small proportion of the admitted patients, resulting in significant errors.

Evaluation and Registration of the Predictive Variables

The next step in the application of a general outcome prediction model is the evaluation, selection, and registration of the predictive variables. At this stage major attention should be given to the variable definitions as well as to the time frames for data collection [37-39]. Often, models have been applied incorrectly, the most common error being related to:
- The definitions of the variables
- The time frames for the evaluation and registration of the data
- The frequency of measurement and registration of the variables
- The applied exclusion criteria
- Data handling before analysis

It should be noted that all existing models have been calibrated for non-automated, i.e. manual data collection. The use of electronic patient data management systems (with high sampling rates) has been demonstrated to have a significant impact on the results [40, 41].

The evaluation of intra and inter-observer reliability should always be described and reported, together with the frequency of missing values.

Evaluation and Registration of the Outcome

All current general outcome prediction models aim to predict the vital status at hospital discharge. It is thus incorrect to use them to predict other outcomes, such as the vital status at ICU discharge. This will result in a gross underestimation of mortality rates [42].

Computation of the Severity Score

Using the original score sheets (or a computer software, well developed and validated), a score is assigned to each variable, depending on its deviation from normal values. The arithmetic sum of these variable scores (the sum score) represents the severity score for that patient, which is then used in the equation to predict hospital mortality. As described above, this approach was not chosen by the authors of the MPM systems, where the variables are directly used to compute a probability of death in the hospital by a logistic regression equation.

Transformation of the Score into a Probability of Death

The transformation of the (severity) score into a probability of death in the hospital uses a logistic regression equation. The dependent variable (hospital mortality) y is related to a set of independent (predictive) variables by the equation:

$$Y = b_0 + b_1 x_1 + b_2 x_2 \ldots b_k x_k$$

with b_0 being the intercept of the model , x_1 to x_k the predictive variables and b_1 to b_k the estimated regression coefficients. The probability of death is then given by:

$$\text{Probability of death} = \frac{e^{\text{logit}}}{1 + e^{\text{logit}}}$$

with the *logit* being y as described before. The logistic transformation included in this equation allows the S-shaped relationship between the two variables to became linear (on the logit scale). In the extremes of the score (very low or very high values) changes in the probability of death are small; for intermediate values, even small changes in the score are associated with very large changes in the probability of death. This ensures that outliers do not influence the prediction too much.

The Validation of the Models

All predictive models developed for outcome prediction need, of course, to be validated, i.e. to demonstrate their ability to predict the outcome under evaluation. Three aspects should be evaluated in this context: The first aspect is the *calibration*, or the degree of correspondence between the predictions of the model and observed results. The second is *discrimination*, or the capability of the model to distinguish observations with a positive outcome from those with a negative outcome. The third is the uniformity-of-fit of the model, i.e. the performance over various subgroups of patients.

The evaluation of the calibration and discrimination has been named *goodness-of-fit*. The evaluation of the performance of the model in major subgroups has been named *uniformity-of-fit*.

Goodness-of-fit. The evaluation of the goodness-of-fit comprises the evaluation of calibration and discrimination in the analysed population.

Calibration evaluates the degree of correspondence between the estimated probabilities of mortality and the actual mortality in the analysed sample. Four methods are usually proposed: observed/estimated (O/E) mortality ratios, Flora's Z score [43], Hosmer-Lemeshow goodness-of-fit tests [44–46] and calibration curves.

Observed/Estimated mortality ratios are computed by dividing the observed mortality (in other words the number of deaths) by the predicted mortality (in other words the sum of the probabilities of mortality of all patients in the sample). In a perfectly calibrated model this value should be one.

Flora's Z score is a statistic that compares the number of survivors observed in the sample with the number of survivors expected according to the model. The difference is then standardised and compared with a normal distribution table [43]. The utilised statistic is:

$$Z = \frac{S - \sum_{i=1}^{\eta} Pi}{\sqrt{\sum_{i=1}^{n} Pi Qi}}$$

with S being the total number of survivors among n patients, Pi the probability of survival estimated by the models for the patient i and Q being 1-Pi or the probability of dead estimated by the model for patient i. This approach is similar to the O/E ratios.

Hosmer-Lemeshow goodness-of-fit tests are two chi-square statistics proposed for the formal evaluation of the calibration of predictive models [44–46]. In the $\hat{H}$ test, patients are classified into 10 groups according to their probabilities of death. Then, a chi-square statistic is used to compare the observed number of deaths and the predicted number of survivors with the observed number of deaths and the observed number of survivors in each of the groups. The formula is:

$$\hat{C}_g - \hat{H}_g = \sum_{i=1}^{g} \frac{(o_i - e_i)^2}{e_i(1 - \bar{\pi}_i)}$$

with g being the number of groups (usually 10), o_l the number of events observed in group l, e_l the number of events expected in the same group and $\bar{\pi}_l$ the mean estimated probability, always in the group l.

The resulting statistic is then compared with a chi-square table with 8 degrees-of-freedom (model development) or 10 degrees-of-freedom (model validation), in order to know if the observed differences can be explained exclusively by random fluctuation. The Hosmer-Lemeshow $\hat{C}$ test is similar, with the 10 groups containing equal number of patients. Hosmer and Lemeshow demonstrated that the grouping method used on the $\hat{C}$ statistics behaves better when most of the probabilities are low [44].

These tests are nowadays considered to be mandatory for the evaluation of calibration [47], although subject to criticism [20, 48]. It should be stressed that the analysed sample must be large enough to have the power to detect the lack of agreement between predicted and observed mortality rates [49].

Calibration curves are also used to describe the calibration of a predictive model. These types of graphics compare observed and predicted mortality. They can be misleading, since the number of patients usually decreases from left to right (when we move from low probabilities to high probabilities) and as a consequence, even small differences in high severity groups appear visually more important than small differences in low probabilities groups. It should be stressed that calibration curves are not a formal statistical test.

Discrimination evaluates the capability of the model to distinguish between patients who die from patients who survive. This evaluation can be made using a non-parametric test such as Harrell's C index, using the order of magnitude of the error [50]. This index measures the probability of, for any two patients chosen randomly, the one with the greater probability to have the outcome of interest (dead). It has been shown that this index is directly related with the area under the receiver operating characteristics (ROC) curve and that it can be obtained as the parameter of the Mann-Whitney-Wilcox statistic [51]. Additional computations can be used to compute the confidence interval of this measure [52].

The concept of the area under the receiver operating characteristic (ROC) curve is derived from psycho-physic tests. In a ROC curve, a series of two by two contingency tables are built, varying from the smallest to the largest score value. For each table the rate of true positive (or sensitivity) and the false-positive rate (or 1 minus the specificity) are calculated. The final plot of all possible pairs of rates of true-positives versus false-positives gives then the visual representation of the ROC curve.

The interpretation of the area under the ROC curve is easy: a virtual model with a perfect discrimination would have an area of 1.0, a model with a discrimination no better than chance an area of 0.5. Discriminative abilities are said to be satisfactory when the ROC curve is > 0.70. General outcome prediction models usually have areas greater than 0.80.

Several methods have been described to compare the areas under two (or more) ROC curves [53–55], but they can be misleading if the shape of the curves is different [56].

Other measures have been utilised based on *classification tables*, wich describe sensitivity, specificity, positive and negative predictive values, and the correct classification rates. However since these calculations must use a fixed cut-off (usually 10, 50 or 90%), their value is limited.

The relative importance of calibration and discrimination depends on the intended use of the model. Some authors advise that for group comparison calibration is especially important [57], and that for decisions involving individual patients both parameters are important [58].

Uniformity-of-Fit

The evaluation of calibration and discrimination in the analysed sample is nowadays current practice. More complex is the identification of sub-groups of patients where the behaviour of the model is non-optimal. These subgroups can be viewed as influential observations in model building and their contribution for the global error of the model can be very large [59].

The most important sub groups are related to the case-mix characteristics that can be eventually related to the outcome of interest, include:
- The intra-hospital location before ICU admission
- The surgical status
- The degree of physiological reserve (age, co-morbidities)
- The acute diagnosis (including infection)

Although some authors, such as Rowan and Goldhill in the United Kingdom [60, 61] and Apolone and Sicignano in Italy [62, 63], have suggested that the behaviour of a model can depend to a significant extent on the case mix of the sample, no consensus exists about the sub-populations that should mandatorily be analysed [64].

Updating the Model

Changes in the characteristics of the populations, changes in the therapy of major diseases, or the introduction of new diagnostic methods all imply modifications that result in necessary updates. Moreover, the use of a model outside its development population can eventually imply its modification and adaptation.

An example of this problem can be found in the results of the EURICUS-I study. The need for accurate estimates of hospital mortality forced the development of new equations for the MPM II_0. It was demonstrated that it was possible to re-calibrate a model by changing all the regression coefficients instead of just changing the relationship between the aggregated score and the outcome of interest. However, some problems in the behaviour of the model in sub-groups remained [65]. A similar strategy was also followed in Austria by Metnitz et al. to adapt SAPS II to the Austrian population [66] and by Rivera-Fernandez and William Knaus to adapt APACHE III to the Spanish population [32].

Such modifications may also be necessary for the application of a general outcome prediction model to a specific population, such as for a patient with sepsis [67–69].

Applicability and Utility of the Model

After validation, the utility and applicability of a model must be evaluated. Literature is full of models developed in large populations that failed, when applied within other contexts [30, 32, 60, 63, 66, 70–72]. Thus, this question can only be answered by validating the model in its final population.

The potential applications of a model – and consequently its utility – are different for individual patients and for groups [73].

Evaluating Individual Patients

Some evidence exists that suggests that statistical methods behave better than clinicians in predicting outcome [74–81], or that they can help clinicians in the decision-making process [82–84]. This opinion is, however, controversial [85–87], especially for decisions to withdraw or to withhold therapy [88]. Moreover, the application of different models to the same patient results frequently in very different predictions [89]. Thus, application of these models to individual patients for decision making is not recommended [90].

It should not be forgotten that such statistical models are of a probabilistic nature. A well-calibrated model, applied to an individual patient may, for example, predict a hospital mortality of 46% for this individual; this, however, just means that for a group of e.g. 100 patients with a similar severity of illness, 46 patients are predicted to die; it makes no statement if the individual patient is included in the 46% who will eventually die or in the 54% that will eventually survive.

It should be noted that severity scores have been proposed for uses as diverse as to determine the use of total parenteral nutrition [91] or the identification of futility in intensive care medicine [92]. Some authors demonstrated that knowledge of predictive information will not have an adverse effect on the quality of care, rather it will help at the same time to decrease the consumption of resources and to increase the availability of beds [93].

One field where the scientific community agrees consensually is the stratification of patients for inclusion into clinical trials and for the comparison of the balance of randomisation in different groups [94].

Group Evaluation

At group level, general outcome prediction models have been proposed for two objectives: distribution of resources and performance evaluation.

Several studies were published describing methods to identify and to characterise patients with a low risk of mortality [95–99]. This type of patient, that requires only basic monitoring and general care, could eventually be transferred to other areas of the hospital [84, 100]. One could, however, also argue that these patients have only a low mortality because they have been monitored and cared for in an ICU [101]. Also, the use of current instruments is not recommended as a triage instrument in the emergency department [102], and also the use of early physiological indicators outside the ICU is being questioned [103].

Moreover, patient costs in the ICU depend on the amount of required (and utilised) nursing workload use. Patient characteristics (diagnosis, degree of physiological dysfunction) are thus not the only determinants: costs depend also on the practices and policies in a given ICU. To focus our attention on the effective use of nursing workload [104] or the dynamic evolution of the patient [27, 105] seems thus a more promising strategy than those approaches based exclusively on the condition of the patients during the first hours in the ICU or in the O/E length of stay in the ICU [106–108].

On the other hand, general outcome prediction models have been proposed to identify patients that require more resources [109]. Unfortunately, these patients only rarely can be identified at ICU admission, since their degree of physiological dysfunction during the first 24 hours in the ICU tends usually to be moderate, although very variable [110–112]. And, even if one day these patients might be well identified, the question of what to do with this information remains.

Another important area where these type of models have been used is in the evaluation of ICU performance. Several investigators proposed the use of standardised mortality ratios (SMR) for performance evaluation, assuming that current models can take into account the main determinants of mortality [113]. The SMR is computed by dividing the observed mortality by the averaged predicted mortality (the sum of the individual probabilities of mortality of all the patients in the sample). Additional computations can be made to estimate the confidence interval of this ratio [114].

The interpretation of the SMR is easy: a ratio lower than one implies a performance better than the reference population, and a ratio greater than one implies a performance worse than the reference population.

This methodology has been used for international comparison of ICUs [3, 60, 71, 115–117], comparison of hospitals [2, 30, 72, 106, 107, 113, 118, 119], ICU evaluation [120–123], management evaluation [119, 124, 125] or the influence of organisation and management factors on the performance of the ICU [126].

Before applying this methodology, six questions should always be answered:
- Can we evaluate and register all the data needed for the computation of the models?
- Can the models be used in the majority of our patients?
- Are existent models able to control for the main patient characteristics related to mortality?
- Has the reference population been well chosen and are the models well calibrated to this population?
- Is the sample size enough to draw meaningful differences?
- Is vital status at ICU discharge the main performance indicator?

Each of these assumptions has been questioned in the last years and there is no definitive answer at this time. However, most investigators believe that performance is multidimensional and consequently that it should be evaluated in several dimensions [127, 128]. The problem of sample size seems especially important with respect to the risk of a type II error (in other words to say that there are no differences when they exist).

Moreover, the comparison between observed and predicted might make more sense if done separately in low-, intermediate-, and high-risk patients, since the performance of an ICU can change according to the severity of the admitted patients. This approach was advocated in the past based on theoretical concerns [129–131], but used only in a short number of studies [126, 132]. Multi-level modelling, with varying slopes, can be an answer for the developers of such models [127, 133].

Conclusions

Over the last few years, outcome prediction has made its way into the ICU as a major scientific discipline. This fact, together with advances in the availability of data and their quality (related mainly to the increasing available computer power) made the introduction of newer statistical methods possible. Also, the first models, using information collected in more regions than

Table 1. General severity scores and outcome prediction models

Characteristics	APACHE	SAPS	APACHE II	MPMᵃ	APACHE III	SAPS II	MPM IIᵇ
Years	1981	1984	1985	1988	1991	1993	1993
Countries	1	1	1	1	1	12	12
ICUs	2	8	13	1	40	137	140
Patients	705	679	5815	2783	17440	12997	19124
Selection of variables and their weights	Panel of experts	Panel of experts	Panel of experts	Multiple logistic regression	Multiple logistic regression	Multiple logistic regression	Multiple logistic regression
Variables:							
Age	No	Yes	Yes	Yes	Yes	Yes	Yes
Origin	No	No	No	No	Yes	No	No
Surgical status	No	No	Yes	Yes	Yes	Yes	Yes
Chronic health status	Yes	No	Yes	Yes	Yes	Yes	Yes
Physiology	Yes	Yes	Yes	Yes	Yes	Yes	Yes
Acute diagnosis	No	No	Yesᶜ	No	Yesᵈ	No	Yes
Number of variables	34	14	17	11	26	17	15ᵉ
Score	Yes	Yes	Yes	No	Yes	Yes	No
Mortality prediction	No	No	Yes	Yes	Yes	Yes	Yes

APACHE Acute Physiology and Chronic Health Evaluation, *SAPS* Simplified Acute Physiology Score, *MPM* Mortality Probability Models
ᵃ These models are based on previous versions, developed by the same authors [134, 135], ᵇThe numbers presented are those for the admission component of the model (MPM II$_0$). MPM II$_{24}$ was developed based on data from 15925 patients from the same ICUs, ᶜchosen from a list of 50 diagnosis, ᵈchosen from a list of 78 diagnosis, ᵉMPM II$_{24}$ uses only 13 variables

Europe and North America, will appear soon. This information should now be combined with dynamic information, with newer models aimed at the prediction of several outcomes and following the physiology of the patient as it is changing. This is the challenge for outcome research.

References

1. Knaus WA, Zimmerman JE, Wagner DP et al (1981) APACHE - acute physiology and chronic health evaluation: a physiologically based classification system. Crit Care Med 9:591–597
2. Knaus WA, Draper EA, Wagner DP et al (1982) Evaluating outcome from intensive care: A preliminary multihospital comparison. Crit Care Med 10:491–496
3. Knaus WA, Le Gall JR, Wagner DP et al (1982) A comparison of intensive care in the U.S.A. and France. Lancet 2:642–646
4. Wagner DP, Draper EA, Abizanda Campos R et al (1984) Initial international use of APACHE: an acute severity of disease measure. Med Decis Making 4:297
5. Le Gall JR, Loirat P, Alperovitch A et al (1984) A Simplified Acute Physiologic Score for ICU patients. Crit Care Med 12:975–977
6. Knaus WA, Draper EA, Wagner DP et al (1985) APACHE II: a severity of disease classification system. Crit Care Med 13:818–829
7. Lemeshow S, Teres D, Avrunin J et al (1988) Refining intensive care unit outcome by using changing probabilities of mortality. Crit Care Med 16:470–477
8. Knaus WA, Wagner DP, Draper EA et al (1991) The APACHE III prognostic system. Risk prediction of hospital mortality for critically ill hospitalized adults. Chest;100:1619–1636
9. Le Gall JR, Lemeshow S, Saulnier F (1993) A new simplified acute physiology score (SAPS II) based on a European/North American multicenter study. JAMA 270:2957–2963
10. Lemeshow S, Teres D, Klar J (1993) Mortality Probability Models (MPM II) based on an international cohort of intensive care unit patients. JAMA 270:2478–2486
11. Castella X, Artigas A, Bion J (1995) The European / North American Severity Study Group. A comparison of severity of illness scoring systems for intensive care unit patients: results of a multicenter, multinational study. Crit Care Med 23:1327–1335
12. Bertolini G, D'Amico R, Apolone G et al (1998) Predicting outcome in the intensive care unit using scoring systems: is new better? A comparison of SAPS and SAPS II in a cohort of 1393 patients. Med Care 36:1371–1382
13. Higgins T, Teres D, Copes W (2005) Preliminary update of the Mortality Prediction Model (MPM0). Crit Care 9:S97 (abs)
14. Render ML, Kim M, Deddens J et al (2005) Variation in outcomeds in Veterans Affairs intensive care units with a computerized severity measure. Crit Care Med 33:930–939
15. Dybowski R, Weller P, Chang R (1996) Prediction of outcome in critically ill patients using artificial neural network, synthesised by genetic algorithm. Lancet 347:1146–1150
16. Engoren M, Moreno R, Reis Miranda D (1999) A genetic algorithm to predict hospital mortality in an ICU population. Crit Care Med 27:A52
17. Ruttimann U, Pollack MM, Fiser DH (1996) Prediction of three outcome states from pediatric intensive care. Crit Care Med 24:78–85

18. Parsonnet V, Dean D, Bernstein A (1989) A method for uniform stratification of risk for evaluating the results of surgery in acquired adult heart disease. Circulation 79:I3-I12

19. Smith EJ, Ward AJ, Smith D (1990) Trauma scoring methods. Br J Hosp Med 44:114–118

20. Champion HR, Copes WS, Sacco WJ et al (1996) Improved predictions from a severity characterization of trauma (ASCOT) over trauma and injury severity score (TRISS): results of an independent evaluation. J Trauma 40:42–49

21. Boyd C, Tolson M, Copes W (1987) Evaluating trauma care: the TRISS method. J Trauma 27:370–378

22. Alberti C, Brun-Buisson C, Chevret S et al (2005) Systemic Inflammatory Response and Progression to Severe Sepsis in Critically Ill Infected Patients. Am J Respir Crit Care Med 171:461–468

23. Vincent J-L, Moreno R, Takala J et al (1996) The SOFA (Sepsis-related organ failure assessment) score to describe organ dysfunction/failure. Intensive Care Med 22:707–710

24. Marshall JD (1997) The multiple organ dysfunction (MOD) score. Sepsis 1:49–52

25. Le Gall J-R, Klar J, Lemeshow S (1997) How to assess organ dysfunction in the intensive care unit? The logistic organ dysfunction (LOD) system. Sepsis 1:45–47

26. Timsit JF, Fosse JP, Troche G et al (2001) Accuracy of a composite score using daily SAPS II and LOD scores for predicting hospital mortality in ICU patients hospitalized for more than 72 h. Intensive Care Med 27:1012–1021

27. Moreno R, Vincent J-L, Matos R et al (1999) The use of maximum SOFA score to quantify organ dysfunction/failure in intensive care. Results of a prospective, multicentre study. Intensive Care Med 25:686–696

28. Bernard GR (1998) Quantification of organ dysfunction: seeking standardization. Crit Care Med 26:1767–1768

29. Boyd O, Grounds M (1994) Can standardized mortality ratio be used to compare quality of intensive care unit performance? Crit Care Med 22:1706–1708

30. Bastos PG, Sun X, Wagner DP (1996) The Brazil APACHE III Study Group. Application of the APACHE III prognostic system in Brazilian intensive care units: a prospective multicenter study. Intensive Care Med 22:564–570

31. Bastos PG, Knaus WA, Zimmerman JE (1996) The Brazil APACHE III Study Group. The importance of technology for achieving superior outcomes from intensive care. Intensive Care Med 22:664–669

32. Rivera-Fernandez R, Vazquez-Mata G, Bravo M et al (1998) The Apache III prognostic system: customized mortality predictions for Spanish ICU patients. Intensive Care Med 24:574–581

33. Cho D-Y, Wang Y-C (1997) Comparison of APACHE III, APACHE II and Glasgow Coma Scale in acute head injury for prediction of mortality and functional outcome. Intensive Care Med 23:77–84

34. Pappachan JV, Millar B, Bennett ED (1999) Comparison of outcome from intensive care admission after adjustment for case mix by the APACHE III prognostic system. Chest 115:802–810

35. Beck DH, Smith GB, Pappachan JV et al (2003) External validation of the SAPS II, APACHE II and APACHE III prognostic models in South England: a multicentre study. Intensive Care Med 29:249–256

36. Lemeshow S, Klar J, Teres D et al (1994) Mortality probability models for patients in the intensive care unit for 48 or 72 hours: a prospective, multicenter study. Crit Care Med 22:1351–1358

37. Abizanda Campos R, Balerdi B, Lopez J et al (1994) Fallos de prediccion de resultados mediante APACHE II. Analisis de los errores de prediction de mortalidad en pacientes criticos. Med Clin Barc 102:527–531

38. Fery-Lemmonier E, Landais P, Kleinknecht D et al (1995) Evaluation of severity scoring systems in the ICUs: translation, conversion and definitions ambiguities as a source of inter-observer variability in APACHE II, SAPS, and OSF. Intensive Care Med 21:356–360

39. Rowan K (1996) The reliability of case mix measurements in intensive care. Curr Opin Crit Care 2:209–213

40. Bosman RJ, Oudemane van Straaten HM, Zandstra DF (1998) The use of intensive care information systems alters outcome prediction. Intensive Care Med 24:953–958

41. Suistomaa M, Kari A, Ruokonen E et al (2000) Sampling rate causes bias in APACHE II and SAPS II scores. Intensive Care Med 26:1773–1778

42. Moreno R, Miranda DR, Matos R et al (2001) Mortality after discharge from intensive care: the impact of organ system failure and nursing workload use at discharge. Intensive Care Med 27:999–1004

43. Flora JD (1978) A method for comparing survival of burn patients to a standard survival curve. J Trauma 18:701–705

44. Hosmer DW, Lemeshow S (1989) Applied logistic regression. New York, John Wiley & Sons, pp

45. Lemeshow S, Hosmer DW (1982) A review of goodness of fit statistics for use in the development of logistic regression models. Am J Epidemiol 115:92–106

46. Hosmer DW, Lemeshow S (1980) A goodness-of-fit test for the multiple logistic regression model. Comm Stat A 10:1043–1069

47. Hadorn DC, Keeler EB, Rogers WH (1993) Assessing the performance of mortality prediction models. Santa Monica, CA, RAND/UCLA/Harvard Center for Health Care Financing Policy Research

48. Bertolini G, D'Amico R, Nardi D (2000) One model, several results: the paradox of the Hosmer-Lemeshow goodness-of-fit test for the logistic regression model. J Epidemiol Biostatistics 5:251–253

49. Zhu B-P, Lemeshow S, Hosmer DW (1996) Factors affecting the performance of the models in the mortality probability model and strategies of customization: a simulation study. Crit Care Med 24:57–63

50. Harrell Jr. FE, Califf RM, Pryor DB (1982) Evaluating the yield of medical tests. JAMA 247:2543–2546

51. Hanley J, McNeil B (1982) The meaning and use of the area under a receiver operating characteristic (ROC) curve. Radiology 143:29–36

52. Ma G, Hall WJ (1993) Confidence bands for receiver operating characteristic curves. Med Decis Making 13:191–197

53. Hanley J, McNeil B (1983) A method of comparing the areas under receiver operating characteristic curves derived from the same cases. Radiology 148:839–843

54. McClish DK (1987) Comparing the areas under more than two independent ROC curves. Med Decis Making 7:149–155

55. DeLong ER, DeLong DM, Clarke-Pearson DL (1988) Comparing the areas under two or more correlated receiver operating characteristic curves: a nonparametric approach. Biometrics 44:837–845

56. Hilden J (1991) The area under the ROC curve and its competitors. Med Decis Making 11:95–101

57. Schuster DP (1992) Predicting outcome after ICU admission. The art and science of assessing risk. Chest 102:1861–1870

58. Kollef MH, Schuster DP (1994) Predicting intensive care unit outcome with scoring systems. Underlying concepts and principles. Crit Care Clin 10:1–18

59. Miller ME, Hui SL (1991) Validation techniques for logistic regression models. Stat Med 10:1213–1226

60. Rowan KM, Kerr JH, Major E et al (1993) Intensive Care Society's APACHE II study in Britain and Ireland - II: Outcome comparisons of intensive care units after adjustment for case mix by the American APACHE II method. Br Med J 307:977–981

61. Goldhill DR, Withington PS (1996) The effects of casemix adjustment on mortality as predicted by APACHE II. Intensive Care Med 22:415–419

62. Sicignano A, Carozzi C, Giudici D et al (1996) The influence of length of stay in the ICU on power of discrimination of a multipurpose severity score (SAPS). Intensive Care Med 22:1048–1051

63. Apolone G, D'Amico R, Bertolini G et al (1996) The performance of SAPS II in a cohort of patients admitted in 99 Italian ICUs: results from the GiViTI. Intensive Care Med 22:1368–1378

64. Moreno R, Apolone G, Reis Miranda D (1998) Evaluation of the uniformity of fit of general outcome prediction models. Intensive Care Med 24:40–47

65. Moreno R, Apolone G (1997) The impact of different customization strategies in the performance of a general severity score. Crit Care Med 25:2001–2008

66. Metnitz PG, Valentin A, Vesely H et al (1999) Prognostic performance and customization of the SAPS II: results of a multicenter Austrian study. Intensive Care Med 25:192–197

67. Knaus WA, Harrell FE, Fisher CJ et al (1993) The clinical evaluation of new drugs for sepsis. A prospective study design based on survival analysis. JAMA 270:1233–1241

68. Le Gall J-R, Lemeshow S, Leleu G et al (1995) Customized probability models for early severe sepsis in adult intensive care patients. JAMA 273:644–650

69. Knaus WA, Harrell FE, LaBrecque JF et al (1996) Use of predicted risk of mortality to evaluate the efficacy of anticytokine therapy in sepsis. Crit Care Med 24:46–56

70. Castella X, Gilabert J, Torner F et al (1991) Mortality prediction models in intensive care: Acute Physiology and Chronic Health Evaluation II and Mortality Prediction Model compared. Crit Care Med 19:191–197

71. Sirio CA, Tajimi K, Tase C et al (1992) An initial comparison of intensive care in Japan and United States. Crit Care Med 20:1207–1215

72. Moreno R, Morais P (1997) Outcome prediction in intensive care: results of a prospective, multicentre, Portuguese study. Intensive Care Med 23:177–186

73. Moreno R (2003) From the evaluation of the individual patient to the evaluation of the ICU. Réanimation 12:47s–48s

74. Perkins HS, Jonsen AR, Epstein WV (1986) Providers as predictors: using outcome predictions in intensive care. Crit Care Med 14:105–110

75. Silverstein MD (1988) Predicting instruments and clinical judgement in critical care. JAMA 260:1758–1759

76. Dawes RM, Faust D, Mechl PE (1989) Clinical versus actuarial judgement. Sci Med Man 243:1674–1688

77. Kleinmuntz B (1990) Why we still use our heads instead of formulas: toward an integrative approach. Psychol Bull 107:296–310

78. McClish DK, Powell SH (1989) How well can physicians estimate mortality in a medical intensive care unit? Med Decis Making 9:125–132

79. Poses RM, Bekes C, Winkler RL et al (1990) Are two (inexperienced) heads better than one (experienced) head? Averaging house officers prognostic judgement for critically ill patients. Arch Intern Med 150:1874–1878

80. Poses RM, Bekes C, Copare FJ et al (1989) The answer to 'what are my chances, doctor?' depends on whom is asked: prognostic disagreement and inaccuracy for critically ill patients. Crit Care Med 17:827–833

81. Winkler RL, Poses RM (1993) Evaluating and combining physicians' probabilities of survival in an intensive care unit. Management science 39:1526–1543

82. Chang RWS, Lee B, Jacobs S et al (1989) Accuracy of decisions to withdraw therapy in critically ill patients: clinical judgement versus a computer model. Crit Care Med 17:1091–1097

83. Knaus WA, Rauss A, Alperovitch A et al (1990) Do objective estimates of chances for survival influence decisions to withhold or withdraw treatment? Med Decis Making 10:163–171

84. Zimmerman JE, Wagner DP, Draper EA et al (1994) Improving intensive care unit discharge decisions: supplementary physician judgment with predictions of next day risk for life support. Crit Care Med 22:1373–1384

85. Branner AL, Godfrey LJ, Goetter WE (1989) Prediction of outcome from critical illness: a comparison of clinical judgement with a prediction rule. Arch Intern Med 149:1083–1086

86. Kruse JA, Thill-Baharozin MC, Carlson RW (1988) Comparison of clinical assessment with APACHE II for predicting mortality risk in patients admitted to a medical intensive care unit. JAMA 260:1739–1742

87. Marks RJ, Simons RS, Blizzard RA et al (1991) Predicting outcome in intensive therapy units - a comparison of APACHE II with subjective assessments. Intensive Care Med 17:159–163

88. Knaus WA, Wagner DP, Lynn J (1991) Short-term mortality predictions for critically ill hospitalized adults: science and ethics. Sci Med Man 254:389–394

89. Lemeshow S, Klar J, Teres D (1995) Outcome prediction for individual intensive care patients: useful, misused, or abused? Intensive Care Med 21:770–776

90. Suter P, Armagandis A, Beaufils F et al (1994) Predicting outcome in ICU patients: consensus conference organized by the ESICM and the SRLF. Intensive Care Med 20:390–397

91. Chang RW, Jacobs S, Lee B (1986) Use of APACHE II severity of disease classification to identify intensive-care-unit patients who would not benefit from total parenteral nutrition. Lancet 1483–1486

92. Atkinson S, Bihari D, Smithies M et al (1994) Identification of futility in intensive care. Lancet 344:1203–1206

93. Murray LS, Teasdale GM, Murray GD et al (1993) Does prediction of outcome alter patient management? Lancet 341:1487–1491

94. Gattinoni L, Brazzi L, Pelosi P et al (1995) A trial of goal orientated hemodynamic therapy in critically ill patients. N Engl J Med 333:1025–1032

95. Henning RJ, McClish D, Daly B et al (1987) Clinical characteristics and resource utilization of ICU patients: implementation for organization of intensive care. Crit Care Med 15:264–269

96. Wagner DP, Knaus WA, Draper EA (1987) Identification of low-risk monitor admissions to medical-surgical ICUs. Chest 92:423–428

97. Wagner DP, Knaus WA, Draper EA et al (1983) Identification of low-risk monitor patients within a medical-surgical ICU. Med Care 21:425–433

98. Zimmerman JE, Wagner DP, Knaus WA et al (1995) The use of risk predictors to identify candidates for intermediate care units. Implications for intensive care unit utilization. Chest;108:490–499

99. Zimmerman JE, Wagner DP, Sun X et al (1996) Planning patient services for inter-

mediate care units: insights based on care for intensive care unit low-risk monitor admissions. Crit Care Med 24:1626–1632

100. Strauss MJ, LoGerfo JP, Yeltatzie JA et al (1986) Rationing of intensive care unit services. An everyday occurrence. JAMA 255:1143–1146

101. Civetta JM, Hudson-Civetta JA, Nelson LD (1990) Evaluation of APACHE II for cost containment and quality assurance. Ann Surg 212:266–276

102. Jones AE, Fitch MT, Kline JA (2005) Operational performance of validated physiologic scoring systems for predicting in-hospital mortality among critically ill emergency department patients. Crit Care Med 33:974–978

103. Hillman K, Chen J, Cretikos M et al; MERIT study investigators (2005) Introduction of the medical emergency team (MET) system: a cluster-randomised controlled trial. Lancet 365:2091–2097

104. Moreno R, Reis Miranda D (1998) Nursing staff in intensive care in Europe. The mismatch between planning and practice. Chest 113:752–758

105. Clermont G, Kaplan V, Moreno R et al (2004) Dynamic microsimulation to model multiple outcomes in cohorts of critically ill patients. Intensive Care Med 30:2237–2244

106. Knaus WA, Wagner DP, Zimmerman JE et al (1993) Variations in mortality and length of stay in Intensive Care Units. Ann Intern Med 118:753–761

107. Zimmerman JE, Shortell SM, Knaus WA et al (1993) Value and cost of teaching hospitals: a prospective, multicenter, inception cohort study. Crit Care Med 21:1432–1442

108. Rapoport J, Teres D, Lemeshow S et al (1994) A method for assessing the clinical performance and cost-effectiveness of intensive care units: a multicenter inception cohort study. Crit Care Med 22:1385–1391

109. Teres D, Rapoport J (1991) Identifying patients with high risk of high cost. Chest 99:530–531

110. Cerra FB, Negro F, Abrams J (1990) APACHE II score does not predict multiple organ failure or mortality in post-operative surgical patients. Arch Surg 125:519–522

111. Rapoport J, Teres D, Lemeshow S et al (1990) Explaining variability of cost using a severity of illness measure for ICU patients. Med Care 28:338–348

112. Oye RK, Bellamy PF (1991) Patterns of resource consumption in medical intensive care. Chest 99:695–689

113. Knaus WA, Draper EA, Wagner DP et al (1986) An evaluation of outcome from intensive care in major medical centers. Ann Intern Med 104:410–418

114. Hosmer DW, Lemeshow S (1995) Confidence interval estimates of an index of quality performance based on logistic regression estimates. Stat Med 14:2161–2172

115. Rapoport J, Teres D, Barnett R et al (1995) A comparison of intensive care unit utilization in Alberta and western Massachusetts. Crit Care Med 23:1336–1346

116. Wong DT, Crofts SL, Gomez M et al (1995) Evaluation of predictive ability of APACHE II system and hospital outcome in Canadian intensive care unit patients. Crit Care Med 23:1177–1183

117. Moreno R, Reis Miranda D, Fidler V et al (1998) Evaluation of two outcome predictors on an independent database. Crit Care Med 26:50–61

118. Le Gall JR, Loirat P, Nicolas F et al (1983) Utilisation d'un indice de gravité dans huit services de réanimation multidisciplinaire. Presse Med 12:1757–1761

119. Zimmerman JE, Rousseau DM, Duffy J et al (1994) Intensive care at two teaching hospitals: an organizational case study. Am J Crit Care 3:129–138

120. Chisakuta AM, Alexander JP (1990) Audit in Intensive Care. The APACHE II classi-

fication of severity of disease. Ulster Med J 59:161–167

121. Marsh HM, Krishan I, Naessens JM et al (1990) Assessment of prediction of mortality by using the APACHE II scoring system in intensive care units. Mayo Clin Proc
65:1549–1557

122. Turner JS, Mudaliar YM, Chang RW et al (1991) Acute physiology and chronic health
evaluation (APACHE II) scoring in a cardiothoracic intensive care unit. Crit Care
Med 19:1266–1269

123. Oh TE, Hutchinson R, Short S et al (1993) Verification of the acute physiology and
chronic health evaluation scoring system in a Hong Kong intensive care unit. Crit
Care Med 21:698–705

124. Zimmerman JE, Shortell SM, Rousseau DM et al (1993) Improving intensive care:
observations based on organizational case studies in nine intensive care units: a
prospective, multicenter study. Crit Care Med 21:1443–1451

125. Shortell SM, Zimmerman JE, Rousseau DM et al (1994) The performance of intensive care units: does good management make a difference? Med Care 32:508–25

126. Reis Miranda D, Ryan DW, Schaufeli WB, Fidler V (eds) (1997) Organization and
management of Intensive Care: a prospective study in 12 European countries.
Berlin, Springer

127. Moreno R, Matos R (2000) The 'new' scores: what problems have been fixed, and
what remain. Curr Opin Crit Care 6:158–165

128. Moreno R, Matos R (2001) New issues in severity scoring: interfacing the ICU and
evaluating it. Curr Opin Crit Care 7:469–474

129. Teres D, Lemeshow S (1993) Using severity measures to describe high performance
intensive care units. Crit Care Clin 9:543–954

130. Teres D, Lemeshow S (1994) Why severity models should be used with caution. Crit
Care Clin 10:93–110

131. Teres D, Lieberman S (1991) Are we ready to regionalize pediatric intensive care?
Crit Care Med 19:139–140

132. Pollack MM, Alexander SR, Clarke N et al (1990) Improved outcomes from tertiary
center pediatric intensive care: a statewide comparison of tertiary and nontertiary
care facilities. Crit Care Med 19:150–159

133. Goldstein H, Spiegelhalter DJ (1996) League tables and their limitations: statistical
issues in comparisons of institutional performance. J R Stat Soc A 159:385–443

134. Lemeshow S, Teres D, Pastides H et al (1985) A method for predicting survival and
mortality of ICU patients using objectively derived weights. Crit Care Med
13:519–525

135. Lemeshow S, Teres D, Avrunin JS et al (1987) A comparison of methods to predict
mortality of intensive care unit patients. Crit Care Med 15:715–722

Clinical Decision Making for Non-Invasive Ventilation

S. Prayag, A. Jahagirdar

Introduction

Ventilatory support which is delivered without establishing an endotracheal airway is called non-invasive ventilation (NIV).

The era of mechanical ventilation (MV) began with the cuirass type of negative pressure non-invasive ventilation. This was widely used in the early twentieth century. The evolution of invasive positive pressure ventilation has come a long way since its introduction during the epidemic of poliomyelitis in Denmark in the 1950s. With the advent of invasive mechanical ventilation, there has been increasing awareness of its complications. Hence attempts are being made to look for alternative methods of positive pressure ventilation.

The use of positive pressure during non-invasive ventilation dates back to the 1930s, when Barach et al. [1] demonstrated that continuous positive airway pressure (CPAP) could be useful in the treatment of acute pulmonary oedema. Non-invasive positive pressure ventilation (NPPV) administered nocturnally - and if needed during the day time - via mouthpiece was used successfully to treat patients with neuromuscular diseases in the early 1960s [2].

In the early 1980s, CPAP delivered through a nasal mask for the treatment of obstructive sleep apnea was described [3].

With the realisation that the patient could tolerate positive pressure delivered through a well fitting nasal mask during sleep, NPPV was developed for the management of chronic nocturnal hypoventilation. In the last two decades the technique has leapt to prominence. As we gained more experience, the indications widened and NPPV became available in many more centres. Thus NPPV has moved from being almost unknown outside a few specialist centres, to becoming an important additional tool in the management of patients with respiratory failure. Although the non-invasive negative pressure ventilation has been making a comeback [4], NIV will be considered equivalent to NPPV for the purpose of this article.

With increasing scope of the use of NIV, many trials have been conducted and its use has been explored not only in critical care units, but also in various other locations like emergency rooms, wards, homes etc.

Since the inappropriate use of any therapeutic modality is not without problems, researchers have started concentrating on controlled trials and evidence to make definitive recommendations for the use of NIV.

Clinical decisions that we need to make at the bedside demand that we answer certain questions with evidence. These questions include:

- Why do we need NIV?
- In which patients should we use NIV?
- Where should we use it?
- When should we use NIV?
- How should we apply it?
- What is the future of this technique?

These basic issues that influence the clinician's decision will be addressed in this article to help the clinician in the appropriate use of this ventilatory modality.

Why Do We Need NIV?

The reasons for promoting NIV include:

- A better understanding of the role of ventilatory pump failure in the indications for mechanical ventilation
- The development of ventilatory modalities able to work in synchrony with the patient
- The extensive recognition of complications associated with endotracheal intubation and invasive mechanical ventilation
- In acute respiratory failure, especially in the chronic obstructive pulmonary disease (COPD) subgroup, a substantial reduction of complications were associated with endotracheal intubation and invasive mechanical ventilation [5]

Several theories have been proposed to explain how NIV works in respiratory failure [6, 7].

We now have a better understanding of the contribution of ventilatory pump failure in the need for mechanical ventilation. As a result, it is possible to say that rest to the fatigued muscles improves respiratory muscle function. During NIV, diaphragmatic electromyographic activity and respiratory muscle work has been shown to be reduced [8, 9].

NIV also improves lung compliance in patients with neuromuscular or chest wall diseases, possibly by re-expanding areas of microatelectasis [10]

When used for nocturnal hypoventilation, NIV prevents the blunting of the central ventilatory drive that occurs with hypercapnia.

Advantages over Endotracheal Intubation and Standard Mechanical Ventilation

Endotracheal intubation is not without problems. The following are the potential benefits of NIV over invasive mechanical ventilation:

- Avoidance of endotracheal intubation
- Decreased incidence of nosocomial pneumonia
- Reduced duration of ventilation
- Decreased need for sedation and paralytics
- Decreased incidence of nosocomial sinusitis
- Better ability to communicate
- Ability to have oral intake
- Preservation of effective cough when administered through nasal mask

In intubated patients there is an increased risk of developing nosocomial pneumonia proportionate to the duration of intubation [10]. Infection is associated with longer intensive care unit (ICU) stay, increased costs and a worse outcome [11].

A prospective epidemiological survey conducted by Guerin et al. [12] has shown that NIV reduces the incidence of nosocomial pneumonias.

This reduction in the incidence of nosocomial infection is a consistent and important – probably the most important – advantage of NIV compared with invasive ventilation [13, 14].

Nosocomial pneumonia is also associated with longer ICU stay, increased costs, and worse outcomes [15]. Therefore, the added benefit of NIV would be the reduction in ICU stay, costs, and outcomes.

In a meta analysis of trials comparing the use of NIV with conventional treatment of respiratory failure in COPD patients, the number of complications associated with NIV were significantly lower, with an overall risk reduction of 68%. Almost all of the excess complications occurred because of intubation, suggesting that avoidance of intubation is the major benefit of NPPV [16].

In Which Patients Should We Use NIV?

There is now a trend towards increasing use of NIV in various situations. It is therefore important to see what the data shows.

Chronic Obstructive Pulmonary Disease

The most well-documented, studied and proven benefit of NIV occurs in patients with acute exacerbation of chronic obstructive pulmonary disease (COPD). It is now well documented that NIV should be the first line intervention in addition to the standard medical care to manage respiratory failure secondary to an acute exacerbation of COPD in all suitable patients [16].

NIV has been described as 'a new standard of care' in patients admitted to hospital with an acute exacerbation of COPD [17].

Patients with haemodynamic instability or impending respiratory arrest require urgent intubation and are not candidates for NIV.

NIV is not currently indicated for patients with initially mild exacerbations of COPD.

In milder patients, NIV may allow respiratory muscle rest but may not improve other clinically important outcomes. However, these patients should be monitored and NIV should be instituted if increasing respiratory distress or respiratory acidosis develops despite standard medical therapy [18].

Predictors of poor outcome in patients of COPD [19, 20] include:
- Low pH
- Pneumonia (consolidation) on chest X-ray
- Low body weight
- Bronchiectasis (excessive secretions)
- High acute physiology and chronic health evaluation (APACHE) scores
- Poor neurological status

Cardiogenic Pulmonary Oedema

Acute cardiogenic pulmonary oedema usually presents with sudden onset of respiratory failure, commonly due to sudden decompensation of chronic heart failure.

NIV has been suggested as a suitable approach in the treatment of acute cardiogenic pulmonary oedema. This is based on pathophysiological findings such as a reduction of left ventricular preload or end diastolic volume with secondary improvement in the left ventricular ejection fraction [21, 22].

The most commonly used technique in cardiogenic pulmonary oedema is continuous positive airway pressure (CPAP). A comparison of CPAP plus standard medical treatment with standard medical therapy alone, showed beneficial outcomes with the use of CPAP. There was a reduced risk of intubation with reduction in hospital mortalities [23].

There has been growing interest, however, in the use of biphasic positive airway pressure (BIPAP) in cardiogenic pulmonary oedema. Trials comparing BIPAP ventilation with standard therapy reveal conflicting results. A study by Masip et al. [24] revealed better oxygenation and a reduced intubation rate but no improvement in mortality. Sharon et al. found an increase in mortality and myocardial ischaemia when compared to high dose of nitrates [25].

A study by Mehta et al. [26] comparing mask CPAP with pressure support plus positive end expiratory pressure (PEEP) with comparable oxygen concentrations also found a greater rate of myocardial infarction (MI) with pressure support and was terminated on interim analysis. It is unclear as to whether the increased incidence of MI was due to ventilatory settings on BIPAP per se or due to any differences in studied groups.

A recent study by Nava et al. [27] found no increased risk of MI with mask pressure support ventilation. The results did not reveal any effect on the overall clinical outcome. However the early use of NIV did show improvement in PaO_2/FiO_2, $PaCO_2$, dyspnoea and respiratory rate. Adverse events including MI were evenly distributed in the two groups [27].

With this important issue now addressed and clarified it may be appropriate to consider the use of BIPAP for cardiogenic pulmonary oedema and better guidelines be derived for its successful application in treating respiratory failure resulting from cardiogenic pulmonary oedema.

Acute Hypoxaemic Respiratory Failure

The rationale for using NIV in patients with acute hypoxaemic respiratory failure (ARF) is not different than for using invasive mechanical ventilation. The final aim is to reduce the work and the cost of breathing by unloading the respiratory muscles and to reduce dyspnoea. This can be achieved effectively with the help of NIV as shown by successfully conducted trials and research.

Early studies in predominantly hypoxaemic patients failed to show the advantage of NIV [28, 29]. However, recent studies have demonstrated that NIV does have a role in some patients. Antonelli et al. [30] compared intubation and conventional mechanical ventilation with NIV in these patients. Improvement in oxygenation was similar with the two modes of support. Patients receiving NIV had significantly lower rates of serious complications and those successfully treated with NIV had shorter ICU stay. One point of concern was the high mortality rate associated in the NIV patients eventually requiring endotracheal intubation. Post hoc subgroup analysis showed that patients with higher severity scores (SAPS > 16) had similar outcomes irrespective of the type of ventilation.

NIV may be indicated in some forms of rapidly reversible hypoxic respiratory failure like status asthmaticus [31]. In these situations supporting the failing respiratory function transiently with NIV may be better than using invasive ventilation. But a direct comparison in this group between invasive ventilation and NIV is lacking.

In a meta-analysis of the trials using NIV in ARF [5], a clear benefit is demonstrated in reducing morbidity and mortality in patients with acute or chronic respiratory failure but the benefit in patients with hypoxemic failure is less clear.

Thus NIV may reduce ICU stays, intubation rates, and complications in patients with hypoxemic respiratory failure but significant tangible results in terms of improved outcomes still remain to be seen.

Acute Respiratory Distress Syndrome

The benefits of NIV have been asserted in patients with acute respiratory insufficiency who require transient ventilatory support until the underlying pathology is resolved. On these lines acute respiratory distress syndrome (ARDS) does seem an unlikely indication. A few studies show promising results in terms of reduction in the rates of intubation and improvement in the survival rates [32–34].

However, these results should be interpreted cautiously and with discretion. The use of NIV for ARDS should be limited to appropriate patients with stable haemodynamics who can be closely monitored and where endotracheal intubation is promptly available.

Severe Community Acquired Pneumonia

The evidence for the use of NIV in respiratory failure following severe community acquired pneumonia is scarce and the results are conflicting. Mortality of ICU admissions due to community acquired pneumonia (CAP) is 22-54% and nearly 58-87% of patients with severe CAP develop hypoxic respiratory failure and require mechanical ventilation [35].

In patients of hypoxic respiratory failure, with or without pneumonia, no difference in responce rate was seen with NIV [36, 37]. A retrospective analysis by Conia et al. found that all patients with pneumonia failed NIV and required endotracheal intubation [38]. Meduri et al. by contrast reported an improvement in gas exchange in more than 75% of patients and avoided intubation in 62% of patients with CAP [31].

A multicentre prospective study revealed better outcomes in terms of reduced need for intubation, reduction in respiratory rate and shortened ICU stay. Subgroup analysis revealed major benefits in patients with COPD having severe community acquired pneumonia [39].

Thus the appropriateness of NIV for respiratory failure following CAP is questionable. But it can still be tried in patients considered appropriate as in a COPD with manageable secretions.

Facilitation of Weaning and Extubation

When patients are considered fit for weaning, a distinction has to be made between the need for an artificial airway and the need for ventilatory support. NIV can be beneficial when weaning has failed but when no artificial airway is required.

Trials conducted for the use of optimal ventilatory mode for successful weaning concluded that regardless of the ventilatory mode, the underlying disease of the patient (especially COPD) was the determinant of the outcome in those patients [40, 41].

The rationale for the use of NIV support to facilitate weaning lies in the ability of NIV to affect the increased workload of respiratory muscles. The additive effects of inspiratory support (IPAP) and end expiratory pressure (EPAP) – to counter balance intrinsic PEEP – are also beneficial [42]. In patients failing spontaneous breathing trials through a T-piece, pressure support ventilation delivered through the endotracheal tube and non-invasively after extubation are equally effective in reducing the work of breathing and improving arterial blood gases [43].

Subsequent to a few observational studies, two randomised controlled trials have been performed to test the effectiveness of NIV in patients who were extubated following failure of the first spontaneous breathing trial [44, 45]. Both studies found that this new approach was successful in maintaining adequate gas exchange and compared with the conventional weaning technique shortened the duration of mechanical ventilation. Nava et al. also showed that NIV reduced ICU stay, incidence of nosocomial pneumonia, and improved survival [44].

Recently, a prospective randomised controlled trial was conducted to asses the efficacy of NIV as a weaning measure [46]. Compared with conventional weaning group, the NIV group had shorter periods of invasive ventilation and ICU stay. Besides, there were decreased requirements of tracheotomy to withdraw ventilation, lower incidence of nosocomial pneumonia and septic shock, and an increased ICU and 90 day survival. The trial was terminated after a planned interim analysis showed significant benefits of NIV. The conventional weaning approach was an independent risk factor of decreased ICU and 90 day survival. Hypercapnia was identified as a marker of poor prognosis during a failed spontaneous breathing trial. The detection of hypercapnia during persistently failed weaning attempts should alert physicians to start measures such as NIV to avert poor outcomes associated with this arterial blood gas finding. Another factor influencing the results of the aforementioned studies is that all patients in the previous two trials and 77% of patients in the later trial had chronic pulmonary disorders causing hypercapnia during weaning failure.

The use of NIV for weaning is a very demanding and challenging application requiring skill and good training. Weaning failure has multiple causes and many factors not strictly related to the ventilator problems may contribute to it [47]. NIV may not be the ultimate solution to the weaning problem, but it may be valuable for certain patients, predominantly those with chronic respiratory disease. There is little information available regarding the role of NIV in weaning patients with respiratory distress due to other causes such as ARDS, or post-surgical complications.

Respiratory Failure Following Extubation

Post-extubation respiratory failure is one of the major problems encountered in an ICU. Following an evidence-based protocol for weaning and discontinuation of mechanical ventilation, the documented need for reintubation ranges from 13 to 19% [40, 48].

Reintubation is an independent risk factor for mortality and nosocomial pneumonia in mechanically ventilated patients. Hospital mortality in patients with extubation failure is up to seven times more than those who are successfully weaned [49–51].

This suggests that the increased mortality seen in these patients may be reduced at least to some extent by treatments aimed at reducing either the need for reintubation or its subsequent complications.

NIV has been deemed by a recent international consensus conference to be a promising therapy after failure of extubation [52]. Subsequently, a randomised controlled trial conducted by Keenan et al. [53] reported no difference in either the rate of intubation or of mortality with the use of NIV as compared with standard medical therapy in patients who have respiratory failure within 48 hours of extubation. It was a small single centre study, hence the extent to which these results can be generalised has been questioned [54].

Further, a multicentre randomised controlled trial evaluated the use of NIV in patients having respiratory failure within 48 hours of extubation [55]. The main finding of this study was that NIV did not reduce mortality or the need for reintubation. The mortality rate tended to be higher among the patients assigned to NIV and the interval from the development of respiratory failure to reintubation was significantly longer with NIV than with standard therapy. The trial was stopped after an interim analysis. The factors that may have influenced the results were the experience of the health care team with NIV, the timing of initiation of NIV after the development of respiratory failure and the composition of the study population. NIV has consistently shown positive results in a patient population who predominantly have chronic respiratory problems. Only 10% of the patients in this study had COPD [55].

Thus, NIV can potentially be effective in averting the need for reintubation in patients developing respiratory failure following extubation but this hypothesis needs to be tested prospectively by conducting further studies.

Post-Operative Respiratory Failure

Thoracic and upper abdominal surgeries are associated with a marked and prolonged post-operative reduction in functional residual capacity (FRC), forced vital capacity (FVC) and PaO_2 which can be reversed by applying NIV. Available literature does suggest the benefit of using NIV in such situations.

Studies conducted by Wysocki et al. and Pennock et al. showed a significant improvement in PaO_2 and a reduction in respiratory rate [56, 57]. NIV was also applied in patients after lung resection surgery with positive results [58].

Other Indications

Antonelli et al. applied NIV in respiratory failure following solid organ transplantation [59]. A sustained improvement in oxygenation was noted along with a significant reduction in the rate of endotracheal intubation, fatal complications, length of ICU stay and ICU mortality.

In patients with cystic fibrosis, mechanical ventilation is commonly associated with dissemination of pulmonary infection and septic shock. Here the avoidance of endotracheal intubation seems crucial with the use of NIV as a bridge to transplantation [60]. Duration of ICU stay and intubation after transplantation were much shorter in this group of patients supported preoperatively with NIV.

Hilbert et al. studied the use of NIV in immunocompromised patients admitted to the ICU for fever, hypoxaemic respiratory failure, and pulmonary infiltrates. NIV significantly reduced the rate of intubation and serious complications [61]. Both ICU and hospital mortality were significantly reduced. Better outcomes were obtained in the subgroup of patients with haematological malignancies and neutropenia suggesting an extended clinical application in these settings [61].

The use of NIV may benefit patients with hypoventilation syndromes like obstructive sleep apnoea or obesity hypoventilation syndrome admitted in ICU for exacerbations. Transient NIV support until the underlying disease resolves may help in stabilising the patient. Proper evidence in these clinical settings is still lacking.

Pulmonary disorders in traumatised patients can be treated with NIV. NIV used in patients with pulmonary contusions or atelectasis showed significant improvement in oxygenation and rates of survival [30]. Gregoretti et al. [62] noted improvement similar to invasive ventilation in gas exchange and respiratory pattern in trauma patients who were given NIV. The recent introduction of the helmet-type masks can make the application of NIV easier in patients with facial or oral trauma who do not tolerate other type of masks.

NIV has been used successfully to overcome the airway resistance caused by laryngeal oedema following extubation [31].

NIV could be used to maintain the patient's comfort, lessen dyspnoea, and permit verbal communication in the group of patients where 'do not intubate' orders have been given. However, this application is controversial with claims that it merely prolongs the dying process leading to inappropriate use of resources.

With larger evidence lacking for the use of NIV in the above mentioned clinical settings, the available results have to be strengthened with more research and evidence. Nevertheless, the option of NIV should be used and explored more enthusiastically by the units actively involved in the treatment of patients with respiratory failure caused by such diverse causes.

Where Should we Use it?

Location

The availability of experienced and skilled clinicians with an equally well trained staff is crucial for the successful implementation of NIV. Hence ICU settings are ideal for NIV in terms of adequacy of staff, good monitoring facilities and rapid access to endotracheal intubation and invasive mechanical ventilation.

With increasing experience, new opportunities regarding the use of NIV outside the ICU location were explored. Subgroup analysis of a multicentre randomised controlled trial of NIV in acute exacerbation of COPD on general respiratory wards in thirteen centres suggested NIV can be applied with benefit outside the ICU after adequate staff trainings [63].

Six prospective randomised controlled studies of NIV outside the ICU show that the timing of initiation of NIV becomes crucial [63–68].

NIV has been shown to be cost-effective both in the ICU and when performed on general wards. A dedicated intermediate care unit with particular expertise in non-invasive modes of ventilation may provide the best environment, both in terms of outcome, and cost-effectiveness.

The ideal location for NIV will vary from country to country and indeed from hospital to hospital, depending upon local factors. However, the most important factor is that staff be adequately trained in the technique and be available throughout the 24 hour period [69].

When Should We Use It?

Absolute contraindications to NIV have been well recognised. These include:
- Cardiopulmonary arrest
- Haemodynamic instability
- Apnoea
- Uncontrolled vomiting
- Gastrointestinal bleeding
- Need for airway protection
- Severely ill patient with multiorgan failure

Apart from the traditional time tested application in COPD, NIV has been successfully tried in other situations like cardiogenic pulmonary oedema, acute hypoxaemic respiratory failure, in immunocompromised patients, in post surgical patients, in facilitation of weaning from mechanical ventilation etc.

Hence the selection of patients becomes a crucial factor for the successful application of NIV. Application of NIV is not without its problems. A high level of vigilance is required to identify those who do not show a response and adherence to defined selection and exclusion criteria should be maintained.

Factors favouring the successful application of NIV [70] are:

- A small volume of respiratory secretions
- The ability to protect the airway
- Synchronous breathing
- Low APACHE scores
- A good initial response in terms of pH, arterial PCO$_2$ and respiratory rate
- Intact dentition

In the patients of COPD, acidosis is an important prognostic factor for survival after respiratory failure. Thus early correction of acidosis, is an essential goal of the treatment. Applying NIV to COPD patients with lesser physiological disturbance, i.e. in whom pH was not very low, resulted in better outcome [63].

In a recent study [71], the risk factors for NIV failure were elucidated. On multivariate analysis the independent predictors of NIV failure were:

- Presence of pneumonia
- High APACHE II score
- Rapid heart rate
- High PaCO$_2$ after 1 hour of NIV

How Should We Apply It?

Equipment for NIV

For the successful application of NIV adapting mechanical ventilation to the patient's needs is critical, as the patient is alert and breathing spontaneously. For nocturnal NIV to be effective, patient comfort without compromising the patient's sleep becomes important. For proper application of NIV therefore, an understanding of the equipment – in particular the ventilators, their modes, and the interface – and its proper selection is mandatory [72].

Ventilators

The smaller portable ventilator used for home ventilation can also be used in the hospitals in ARF. But critical care ventilators continue to be the predominant machines in ICU for NIV. The non availability of pressure-flow wave forms in the portable ventilators is the major limitation for its use. These are important especially in the initial hours of ventilation when it is important to assess the patient/ventilator interaction, respiratory mechanics, and expired tidal volume [73].

Moreover, differences in terms of CO_2 rebreathing, speed of attainment of stable pressure support level and expiratory resistance were found between the critical care and portable ventilators [74].

Volume Targeted Ventilators vs. Pressure Targeted Ventilators

Volume cycled NIV delivers a set volume for each breath. It has been shown to improve outcomes in acute respiratory failure [37]. Compared with pressure ventilators, it is rarely used. A patient's tolerance of this therapy is often poor [75] because of the high inspiratory pressure that may be reached causing leaks and discomfort to the patient [76].

Fluctuation in pressure may increase leakage due to the higher inspiratory pressure reached. Tightening of straps done to minimise leaks may lead to pressure sores or skin necrosis.

Pressure targeted ventilation is the preferred mode in the treatment of ARF [77]. These ventilators have better leak compensating abilities.

In a long-term case study of 30 patients who needed NIV, the authors concluded that in a subpopulation with a clinically stable chronic respiratory failure, volume ventilation may be superior to pressure ventilation [78]. At the end of the study, the majority of patients with equal efficacy of both ventilation modes, preferred pressure-targeted modes as the definitive mode for long term mechanical ventilation for reasons of comfort.

The pressure targeted breaths may be given as CPAP or BIPAP.

Mode

Continuous Positive Airway Pressure (CPAP). By delivering a constant pressure during both inspiration and expiration, it influences breathing mechanics.

In patients with cardiogenic pulmonary oedema, it improves shunt fraction and reduces the work of breathing [79]. In patients with COPD, CPAP works by counterbalancing the inspiratory threshold load when there is intrinsic PEEP [80]. CPAP has also been useful in ARF due to a variety of other aetiologies [23, 81].

Biphasic Positive Airway Pressure (BIPAP). This is commonly given with standard ventilators that use pressure support or pressure control and PEEP in a non-invasive mode. As indicated earlier, the utility of BIPAP in patients of cardiogenic pulmonary oedema has been studied and questioned [24, 26, 27].

Proportional Assist ventilation (PAV). This new modality has been proposed for its properties of synchronised partial ventilatory support. Some studies have already been done [82, 83]. Despite its incorporation in the machine, it currently remains an experimental mode and its clinical impact has not been established [72].

Interface

Another important issue during the setting up of NIV is the choice of optimal interface.
Different types of interfaces are available:
- Full face masks (enclose mouth and nose)
- Nasal mask
- Nasal pillows or plugs
- Mouthpieces
- Custom fabricated masks
- Helmet type

A review of the studies published showed that in ARF, NIV facial masks predominates (63%) followed by nasal masks (31%). In chronic respiratory failure, nasal masks are most commonly used (73%) followed by nasal pillows (11%), facial mask (6%) and mouthpieces (5%) [72]. In ARF a full face mask is chosen in the initial acute phase when mouth breathing is significant. Moreover, studies have found better quality of blood gases and minute ventilation in the initial phase [84, 85].

Helmet masks are now becoming very popular especially with studies showing its efficacy [86].

What is the Future of this Technique?

Since its introduction, NIV has been used increasingly for different clinical situations. New evidence is accumulating as trials are being conducted. It is increasingly clear that even in indications such as COPD, where the maximum benefit of this modality has been shown, there are certain subgroups which will benefit the most, for example the group of patients who are not obtunded severely, whose APACHE score is not too high, whose haemodynamics is not too compromised or those who do not have such severe acidosis. All these would indicate that the subgroup which is severely ill is not likely to benefit from NIV. It is the subgroup which requires mechanical ventilation but whose respiratory failure is only moderately severe, who are more likely to benefit from NIV. Moving away from COPD, benefit from NIV is reported in some patients having respiratory failure due to other indications, again in those not so severely ill. The role of NIV in off loading the respiratory muscles and reducing work of breathing has been proven.

We will, in future, approach NIV with a lot of interest. The interest will be due to its proven benefits in reducing incidence of infections, ICU and hospital length of stay, cost and mortality. Certain subgroups of patients irrespective of aetiology have shown benefits from NIV. Perhaps NIV will become the agent of choice in mild to moderately severe respiratory failure, irrespective of aetiology – if there are no contraindications.

Many believe that with patients who have acute respiratory distress there is a fairly narrow window of opportunity for the use of non-invasive ventilation; they need to be sick enough for intervention but not sick enough to require immediate intubation. The initial six-to-eight-hour period of non-invasive ventilation is resource-intensive, and failure to intubate a patient who does not have a response is associated with increased mortality [87].

The era of NIV has already begun, the future will throw a lot of light on its exact role in the management of critically ill patients.

References

1. Barach AL, Martin J, Eckman M (1938) Positive pressure respiration and its application to treatment of acute pulmonary oedema. Ann Intern Med 12: 754–795
2. Alba A, Khan A, Lee M (1984) Mouth IPPV for sleep. Rehabilitation Gazette 24:47–49
3. Sullivan CE, Berthon-Jones M, Issa FG (1983) Reversal of obstructive sleep apnoea by continuous positive airway pressure applied through the nares. Lancet 321:862
4. Hill NS (2004) Is there still a negative side to non invasive ventilation? Eur Respir J 23:419–424
5. Peter JV, Moran JL, Phillips-Hughes J et al (2002) Noninvasive ventilation in acute respiratory failure. A meta-analysis update. Crit Care Med 30:555–562
6. Claman DM, Piper A, Sanders MH et al (1996) Nocturnal noninvasive positive pressure ventilatory assistance. Chest 110:1581–1588
7. Hill NS (1993) Noninvasive ventilation: does it work, for whom, and how? Am Rev Respir Dis 147:1050–1055
8. Brochard L, Isabey D, Piquet J et al (1990) Reversal of acute exacerbations of chronic obstructive lung disease by inspiratory assistance with a face mask. N Engl J Med 323:1523–1530
9. Renston JP, Di Marco AF, Supinski GS (1994) Respiratory muscle rest using nasal BiPAP ventilation in patients with stable severe COPD. Chest 105:1053–1060
10. Fagon JY, Chastre J, Hance A et al (1993) Nosocomial pneumonia in ventilated patients: a cohort study evaluating attributable mortality and hospital stay. Am J Med 94:281–287
11. Bergofsky EH (1979) Respiratory failure in disorders of the thoracic cage. Am Rev Respir Dis 119:643–669
12. Guerin C, Girard R, Chemorin C et al (1997) Facial mask noninvasive mechanical ventilation reduces the incidence of nosocomial pneumonia. A prospective epidemiological survey from a single ICU. Intensive Care Med 23:1024–1032
13. Nourdine K, Combes P, Carton MJ et al (1999) Does noninvasive ventilation reduce the ICU nosocomial infection risk? A prospective clinical survey. Intensive Care Med 25:567–573

14. Girou E, Schortgen F, Delclaux C et al (2000) Association of noninvasive ventilation with nosocomial infections and survival in critically ill patients. JAMA 284:2361–2367
15. Torres A, Aznar R, Gatell JM et al (1990) Incidence, risk and prognosis factors of nosocomial pneumonia in mechanically ventilated patients. Am Rev Respir Dis 142:523–528
16. Lightowler JV, Wedzicha JA, Elliott MW (2003) Non-invasive positive pressure ventilation to treat respiratory failure resulting from exacerbations of chronic obstructive pulmonary disease: Cochrane systematic review and meta-analysis. BMJ 326:185
17. Brochard L (2000) Non-invasive ventilation for acute exacerbations of COPD: a new standard of care. Thorax 55:817–818
18. Keenan SP, Sinuff T, Cook DJ et al (2003) Which patients with acute exacerbation of chronic obstructive pulmonary disease benefit from noninvasive positive-pressure ventilation? A systematic review of the literature. Ann Intern Med 138:861–870
19. Ambrosino N, Foglio K, Rubini F et al (1995) Non-invasive mechanical ventilation in acute respiratory failure due to chronic obstructive pulmonary disease: correlates for success. Thorax 50:755–757
20. Hill NS (1995) Long term Nasal Ventilation. Thorax 50:595–596
21. Lenique F, Habis M, Lofaso F et al (1997) Ventilatory and hemodynamic effects of continuous positive airway pressure in left heart failure. Am J Respir Crit Care Med 155:500–505
22. Chadda K, Annane D, Hart N et al (2002) Cardiac and respiratory effects of continuous positive airway pressure and noninvasive ventilation in acute cardiac pulmonary edema. Crit Care Med 30:2457–2461
23. Pang D, Keenan SP, Cook DJ et al (1998) The effect of positive pressure airway support on mortality and the need for intubation in cardiogenic pulmonary edema: a systematic review. Chest 114:1185–1192
24. Masip J, Betbes AJ, Vecilla F et al (2000) Non-invasive pressure support ventilation versus conventional oxygen therapy in acute cardiogenic pulmonary edema: a randomised trial. Lancet 356:2126–2132
25. Sharon A, Shpirer I, Kaluski E et al (2000) High-dose intravenous isosorbide-dinitrate is safer and better than Bi-PAP ventilation combined with conventional treatment for severe pulmonary edema. J Am Coll Cardiol 36:832–837
26. Mehta S, Jay GD, Woolard RH et al (1997) Randomized, prospective trial of bilevel versus continuous positive airway pressure in acute pulmonary oedema. Crit Care Med 25:620–628
27. Nava S, Carbone G, Di Battista N et al (2003) Noninvasive ventilation in cardiogenic pulmonary edema: a multicenter randomized trial. Am J of Respir Crit Care Med 168:1432–1437
28 Wysocki M, Tric L, Wolff MA et al (1995) Noninvasive pressure support ventilation in patients with acute respiratory failure. A randomized comparison with conventional therapy. Chest 107:761–768
29. Wood KA, Lewis L, Von Harz B et al (1998) The use of noninvasive positive pressure ventilation in the Emergency Department. Chest 113:1339–1346
30. Antonelli M, Conti G, Rocco M et al (1998) A comparison of noninvasive positive-pressure ventilation and conventional mechanical ventilation in patients with acute respiratory failure. N Engl J Med 339:429–435
31. Meduri GU, Turner RE, Abou-Shala N et al (1996) Noninvasive positive pressure ventilation via face mask. First-line intervention in patients with acute hypercapnic

and hypoxemic respiratory failure. Chest109:179–193

32. Rocker GM, Mackenzie MG, Williams B et al (1999) Noninvasive positive pressure ventilation. Successful outcome in patients with acute lung injury/ARDS. Chest 115:173–177

33. Wysocki M, Vincent JL (1998) Noninvasive ventilation in acute respiratory failure: Technological issues. In: Vincent JL (ed) Yearbook of Intensive Care and Emergency Medicine, Berlin, Springer, pp 519–527

34. Ambrosino N (1996) Noninvasive mechanical ventilation in acute respiratory failure. Eur Respir J 9:795–807

35. Wysocki M, Antonelli M (2001) Non invasive mechanical ventilation in acute hypoxemic respiratory failure. Eur Respir J 18:209–220

36. Pennock BE, Kaplan PD, Carlin BW et al (1991) Pressure support ventilation with a simplified ventilatory support system administered with a nasal mask in patients with respiratory failure. Chest 100:1371–1376

37. Benhamou D, Girault C, Faure C et al (1992) Nasal mask ventilation in acute respiratory failure. Experience in elderly patients. Chest 102:912–917

38. Conia A, Wysocki M, Wolff MA et al (1996) Noninvasive pressure support ventilation for acute respiratory failure in patients with formerly healthy lungs. Feasibility and possible indications. JEUR 91:11–19

39. Confalonieri M, Potena A, Carbone G et al (1999) Acute respiratory failure in patients with severe community-acquired pneumonia. A prospective randomized evaluation of noninvasive ventilation. Am J Respir Crit Care Med 160:1585–1591

40. Esteban A, Frutos F, Tobin MJ et al (1995) A comparison of four methods of weaning patients from mechanical ventilation. N Engl J Med 323:345–350

41. Brochard L, Rauss A, Benito S et al (1994) Comparison of three methods of gradual withdrawal from ventilatory support during weaning from mechanical ventilation. Am J Respir Crit Care Med 150:896–903

42. Appendini L, Patessio A, Zanaboni S et al (1994) Physiologic effects of positive end-expiratory pressure and mask pressure support during exacerbations of chronic obstructive pulmonary disease. Am J Respir Crit Care Med 149:1069–1076

43. Vitacca M, Ambrosino N, Clini E et al (2001) Physiologic response to pressure support ventilation delivered before and after extubation in patients not capable of totally spontaneous autonomous breathing. Am J Respir Crit Care Med 164:638–641

44. Nava S, Ambrosino N, Clini E et al (1998) Noninvasive mechanical ventilation in the weaning of patients with respiration failure due to chronic obstructive pulmonary disease: a randomized, controlled trial. Ann Intern Med 128:721–728

45. Girault C, Daudenthun I, Chevron V et al (1999) Noninvasive ventilation as a systematic extubation and weaning technique in acute-on-chronic respiratory failure: a prospective, randomized controlled study. Am J Respir Crit Care Med 160:86–92

46. Ferrer M, Esquinas A, Arancibia F et al (2003) Noninvasive ventilation during persistent weaning failure: a randomized controlled trial. Am J Respir Crit Care Med 168:70–76

47. Manthous CA, Schmidt GA, Hall JB (1998) Liberation from mechanical ventilation: a decade of progress. Chest 114:886–901

48. Esteban A, Alía I, Tobin MJ et al (1999) Effect of spontaneous breathing trial duration on outcome of attempts to discontinue mechanical ventilation. Am J Respir Crit Care Med 159:512–518

49. Epstein SK, Ciubotaru RL, Wong J (1997) Effect of failed extubation on the outcome of mechanical ventilation. Chest 112:186–192

50. Torres A, Gatell JM, Aznar E et al (1995) Re-intubation increases the risk of nosoco-

mial pneumonia in patients needing mechanical ventilation. Am J Respir Crit Care Med 152:137–141

51. Epstein SK, Ciubotaru RL (1998) Independent effects of etiology of failure and time of reintubation on outcome for patients failing extubation. Am J Respir Crit Care Med 158:489–493

52. Anonymous (2001) International Consensus Conferences in Intensive Care Medicine: non-invasive positive pressure ventilation in acute respiratory failure. Am J Respir Crit Care Med 163:283–291

53. Keenan SP, Powers C, McCormack DG et al (2002) Noninvasive positive-pressure ventilation for postextubation respiratory distress: a randomized controlled trial. JAMA 287:3238–3244

54. Girault C, Auriant I (2002) Differences in success rates of Non invasive ventilation. JAMA 288:2540–2540

55. Esteban A, Frutos-Vivar F, Niall D et al (2004) Noninvasive positive-pressure ventilation for respiratory failure after extubation. N Engl J Med 350:2452–2460

56. Wysocki M, Tric L, Wolff MA et al (1993) Noninvasive pressure support ventilation in patients with acute respiratory failure. Chest 103:907–913

57. Pennock BE, Kaplan PD, Carlin BW et al (1991) Pressure support ventilation with a simplified ventilatory support system administered with a nasal mask in patients with respiratory failure. Chest 100:1371–1376

58. Aguilo R, Togores B, Pons S et al (1997) Noninvasive ventilatory support after lung resectional surgery. Chest 112:117–121

59. Antonelli M, Conti G, Bufi M et al (2000) Noninvasive ventilation for the treatment of acute respiratory failure in patients undergoing solid organ transplantation. JAMA 283:235–241

60. Hodson ME, Madden BP, Steven MH et al (1991) Non-invasive mechanical ventilation for cystic fibrosis patients: a potential bridge to transplantation. Eur Respir J 4:524–527

61. Hilbert G, Gruson D, Vargas F et al (2001) Noninvasive ventilation in immunosuppressed patients with pulmonary infiltrates, fever, and acute respiratory failure. N Engl J Med 344:481–487

62. Gregoretti C, Beltrame F, Lucangelo U et al (1998) Physiologic evaluation of non-invasive pressure support ventilation in trauma patients with acute respiratory failure. Intensive Care Med 24:785–790

63. Plant PK, Owen JL, Elliott MW (2000) Early use of non-invasive ventilation for acute exacerbations of chronic obstructive pulmonary disease on general respiratory wards: a multicentre randomised controlled trial. Lancet 355:1931–1935

64. Bott J, Carroll MP, Conway JH et al (1993) Randomised controlled trial of nasal ventilation in acute ventilatory failure due to chronic obstructive airways disease. Lancet 341:1555–1557

65. Barbe F, Togores B, Rubi M et al (1996) Noninvasive ventilatory support does not facilitate recovery from acute respiratory failure in chronic obstructive pulmonary disease. Eur Respir J 9:1240–1245

66. Angus RM, Ahmed AA, Fenwick LJ et al (1996) Comparison of the acute effects on gas exchange of nasal ventilation and doxapram in exacerbations of chronic obstructive pulmonary disease. Thorax 51:1048–1050

67. Wood KA, Lewis L, Von Harz B et al (1998) The use of noninvasive positive pressure ventilation in the Emergency Department. Chest 113:1339–1346

68. Bardi G, Pierotello R, Desideri M et al (2000) Nasal ventilation in COPD exacerbations: early and late results of a prospective, controlled study. Eur Respir J 15:98–104

69. Elliott MW, Confalonieri M, Nava S (2002) Where to perform noninvasive ventilation? Eur Respir J 19:1159–1166
70. Liesching T, Kwok H, Hill NS (2003) Acute applications of noninvasive positive pressure ventilation. Chest 124:699–713
71. Phua J, KienKong K, Lee KH et al (2005) Noninvasive ventilation in hypercapnic acute respiratory failure due to chronic obstructive pulmonary disease vs. other conditions: effectiveness and predictors of failure. Intensive Care Med 31:533–539
72. Schönhofer B, Sortor-Leger S (2002) Equipment needs for noninvasive mechanical ventilation: Eur Respir J 20:1029–1036
73. Calderini E, Confalonieri M, Puccio PG et al (1999) Patient-ventilator asynchrony during noninvasive ventilation: the role of expiratory trigger. Intensive Care Med 25:662–667
74. Lofaso F, Brochard L, Hang T et al (1996) Home versus intensive care pressure support devices. Experimental and clinical comparison. Am J Respir Crit Care Med 153:1591–1599
75. Foglio C, Vitacca M, Quadri A et al (1992) Acute exacerbations in severe COLD patients: treatment using positive pressure ventilation by nasal mask. Chest 101:1533–1538
76. Soo Hoo GW, Santiago S, Williams AJ (1994) Nasal mechanical ventilation for hypercapnic respiratory failure in chronic obstructive pulmonary disease: determinants of success and failure. Crit Care Med 22:1253–1261
77. Carlucci A, Richard JC, Wysocki M et al (2001) Noninvasive versus conventional mechanical ventilation. An epidemiologic survey. Am J Respir Crit Care Med 163:874–880
78. Schonhofer B, Sonneborn M, Haidl P et al (1997) Comparison of two different modes for noninvasive mechanical ventilation in chronic respiratory failure: volume versus pressure controlled device. Euro Respir J 10:184–191
79. Lin M, Yang YF, Chiang HT et al (1995) Reappraisal of continuous positive airway pressure therapy in acute cardiogenic pulmonary edema. Short-term results and long-term follow-up. Chest 107:1379–1386
80. Petrof BJ, Legare M, Goldberg P et al (1990) Continuous positive airway pressure reduces work of breathing and dyspnea during weaning from mechanical ventilation in severe chronic obstructive pulmonary disease. Am Rev Respir Dis 141:281–290
81. Delclaux C, L'Her E, Alberti C et al (2000) Treatment of acute hypoxemic nonhypercapnic respiratory insufficiency with continuous positive airway pressure delivered by a face mask: A randomized controlled trial. JAMA 284:2352–2360
82. Gay PC, Hess DR, Hill NS (2001) Noninvasive proportional assist ventilation for acute respiratory insufficiency: Comparison with pressure support ventilation. Am J Respir Crit Care Med 164:1606–1611
83. Wysocki M, Richard JC, Meshaka MD (2002) Nonivasive proportional assist ventilation compared with noninvasive pressure support ventilation in hypercapnic acute respiratory failure. Crit Care Med 30:323–329
84. Navalesi P, Fanfulla F, Firgerio P (2000) Physiologic evaluation of noninvasive mechanical ventilation delivered with three types of masks in patients with chronic hypercapnic respiratory failure. Crit Care Med 28:1785–1790
85. Brochard L (2000) What is really important to make noninvasive ventilation work. Crit Care Med 28:2139–2140
86. Antonelli M, Pennisi MA, Pelosi P et al (2004) Noninvasive positive pressure ventilation using a helmet in patients with acute exacerbation of chronic obstructive pul-

monary disease: a feasibility study. Anesthesiology 100:16–24
87. Truwit JD, Bernard GR (2004) Noninvasive Ventilation – Don't Push Too Hard. New Eng J Med 350:2512–2515

Control of Infections in Intensive Care Units

J. Takezawa

Nosocomial Infections in Intensive Care Units (ICUs)

Nosocomial infections are believed to occur most frequently in intensive care units (ICUs), and they affect the outcome of the patients admitted to the ICU. However, this notion was based on CDC/NNIS findings on their overall hospital surveillance of US hospitals in 1970-1990. This notion is, however, still true as far as the use of medical equipments concerned as an external risk factor for developing nosocomial infections. Because ICU is the place where medical equipment is most frequently used in the hospital, the number of the patients who acquire nosocomial infections becomes largest. This is the reason why ICUs became the target of nosocomial infection surveillance in the NNIS system. However, it does not mean that the strength of prevention of nosocomial infections in ICUs is inferior to that of other wards (in order to measure the performance of nosocomial infections preventing capability, infection rates should be calculated while risk adjustment is made). Nevertheless, the incidence of nosocomial infections is highest in ICUs. Therefore, strict preventive measures should be provided to improve the prognosis of the patients.

It is usually believed that because ICUs are the place where most severely ill patients are admitted, they are likely to acquire nosocomial infections. However, this concept is not verified, because the effect of internal risk factors such as the severity of illness on the development of nosocomial infections is not thoroughly evaluated. It can be easily assumed that the most severely ill patients die earlier and therefore are not associated with the development of nosocomial infections as there is no time to acquire nosocomial infections, and the least severely ill patients may be discharged earlier, and so again have no time to acquire nosocomial infections. Therefore, it is unknown whether the severity of illness becomes an internal risk factor for acquiring nosocomial infections in ICUs. In other words, although severity of illness is strongly related to the mortality (as it was originally made for this purpose), it is unknown whether severity of illness is associated with the development of nosocomial infections in ICUs.

Factors for the ICU-Acquired Infection

Several factors are considered to be associated with the development of noso-comial infections in the ICU (Table 1). Among them, indwelling devices that directly come into contact with blood and the mucosal membrane such as a central venous catheter, urinary tract catheter and endotracheal tube; these are considered to be the most important risk factors in the development of nosocomial infections. These devices are placed within the patient and manipulated by the medical practitioner, and are referred to as external risk factors. These device-related external risk factors are associated with the length of exposure to the device. However, they are also associated with the frequency of manipulations of the device, such as bolus injection and exchanges of the infusion bottles and lines, especially for the indwelling CV catheter. In addition to the length and/or frequency of exposure to the risk device, hygienic management, the behaviour pattern of antibiotic adminis-tration and patient management (therapeutic, nursing, monitoring, staffing, and organisational) also become external risk factors in the development of nosocomial infections. On the other hand, the risk factor inherent within the patient is referred to as an internal risk factor and this includes age, gender, severity of illness, immunological competence, comorbidity. These internal risk factors are inherent within the patients, and they cannot be manipulated.

In order to accomplish an inter-institutional comparison on infection rates, both internal and external risk factors need to be adjusted. Among the risk factors indicated above, the internal risk related to severity of illness may be adjusted by using the APACHE scoring system, and the external risk can

Table 1. Risk factors in ICU-acquired infections

Risk	
Internal risk	Age, Gender, Original disease, Severity of illness, Comorbid disease
External risk	Device: CV catheter, Ventilator, Urinary tract catheter Drug: Antibiotics, immunosuppressive drugs Intervention/Operation Infection Control: Hygienic procedures, Manuals, Surveillance
Education	Therapeutic and nursing capability Monitoring capability Organisational characteristics: Open/Closed, Staffing

only be adjusted by device utilisation days. Therefore, the difference in infection rates adjusted by the above two risk factors is attributable to the other remaining external risk factors, most of which are related to the institutional characteristics such as patient and ICU management.

Purpose of Surveillance

The purpose of the surveillance is 1) to identify the outbreak of nosocomial infections (an outbreak is easily noted by ICU practitioners); 2) to indicate the numbers for infection control to be pursued by ICU practitioners for quality improvement; 3) to obtain the incidence and prevalence of nosocomial infections from the viewpoint of public health; 4) to provide inter-institutional comparisons to demarcate preventive programmes and practice of nosocomial infections by the participating institutes.

When surveillance is conducted for the purpose of inter-institutional comparison of the nosocomial infection rate, all risk factors for ICU-acquired infections should be adjusted. The national nosocomial infection surveillance (NNIS) system, which is run by the Centres for Disease Control (CDC), apparently uses only external risk-adjusted infection rate for inter-institutional comparison. The severity of illness in NNIS is ignored and instead, they adopt device utilisation ratio, which is calculated as length of days devices are used, divided by patient days. It is based on the assumption that the severely ill patient requires long-term use of the devices for efficient and safer management. However, the device utilisation ratio as well as APACHE and SAPS scoring systems which are frequently used for stratifying the severity of illness in terms of mortality are not proven to be related to the acquisition of nosocomial infections in the ICU (because the most severely ill patients die quickly), even though the patients who die within 24 hours after admission to the ICU are excluded for inter-hospital comparison of the performance of ICUs in APACHE scoring system.

In the NNIS system, risk-adjusted infection rate is compared within the individual types of ICUs such as neonatal ICU, cardiac care unit, and surgical ICU, which implies that original disease is taken into account as an internal risk factor. However, because all the internal risk factors are not included in the NNIS system, the exact effect of severity of illness on ICU-acquired infections is unknown.

ICU-Acquired Infection and Hospital Mortality

Although the incidence of ICU-acquired infection is known to be one of the important determinants for the outcome of ICU patients, the precise relationship between ICU-acquired infection and hospital mortality has yet to be defined. A 1-day point-prevalence study for 1417 ICUs from 17 Western European countries, known as the EPIC study, showed that a prevalence rate of infection in ICUs was 44.8%, and almost half of the infections were acquired in the ICU (20.6%) [1]. The EPIC study showed that the impact of ICU-acquired infection on ICU mortality might vary according to the types of infection; the highest odds ratio was found in sepsis (3.50), followed by pneumonia (1.91) and blood stream infection (1.73). Moreover, several studies showed that inadequate treatment of infections might be an important determinant of hospital mortality [2, 3].

There have been few cohort studies in which the patients discharged from the ICU were followed up until hospital discharge. One cohort study involving 28 ICUs from 8 countries showed that the hospital mortality rate in patients with ICU-acquired infection was 32.1% against 12.1% of that in patients without ICU-acquired infections [4]. These rates were crude and not adjusted for potential confounders (e.g. age, underlying disease, and severity of illness) [5, 6]. Moreover, the impact of ICU-acquired infection on hospital mortality might be affected by drug-resistant pathogens [7].

JANIS Database Analysis

The Japanese Nosocomial Infection Surveillance (JANIS) system, started in 2000 by the Ministry of Health, Labour, and Welfare, collected the data from 7374 patients admitted to the 34 participating ICUs between July 2000 and May 2002. The data used for their analysis came from patients discharged from ICU aged 16 years or older, whose ICU stay was from 48 to 1000 hours, who had not transferred to another ICU, and who had no infection diagnosed within 2 days after ICU admission, and were followed up until hospital discharge or the 180 day after ICU discharge. Adjusted hazard ratios (HRs) with their 95% confidence intervals (CIs) for hospital mortality were calculated using a Cox's proportional hazard model [8].

Table 2 shows the effect of ICU-acquired infections on hospital mortality. Overall, 678 patients (9.2%) had at least one ICU-acquired infection. Drug-resistant pathogens were detected in 201 patients. The most common ICU-acquired infections were VAP (517 cases, 64%), followed by sepsis (106 cases, 13%), SSI (102 cases, 13%), UTI (43 cases, 5%), and CR-BSI (42 cases, 5%). All types of ICU-acquired infections were significantly associated with hospital mortality. Compared to patients who had no infection, those infected by both drug-susceptible and resistant pathogens showed significantly higher rates of hospital mortality (shown as p-value). The mortality rate from drug-resistant pathogens was higher than that from drug-susceptible pathogens, except for

Table 2. The effect of ICU-acquired infections on hospital mortality

	no. of pts	drug-susceptible	drug-resistant	p-value
VAP				
Alive	5756	230	84	
Deceased	1101	140	63	
% of deceased	16.1	37.8	42.9	< 0.001
UTI				
Alive	6042	25	3	
Deceased	1289	15	0	
% of deceased	17.6	37.5	0	< 0.01
CR-BSI				
Alive	6049	18	3	
Deceased	1277	18	3	
% of deceased	17.4	50.0	50.0	< 0.001
Sepsis				
Alive	6038	24	8	
Deceased	1230	52	22	
% of deceased	16.9	68.4	73.3	< 0.001
SSI				
Alive	6009	44	17	
Deceased	1263	28	13	
% of deceased	17.4	38.9	43.3	< 0.001

VAP ventilator associated pneumonia, *UTI* urinary catheter related infection, *CR-BIS* catheter-related blood stream infection, *SSI* surgical site infection. The total numbers of the patients are different among the ICU-acquired infections because of a lack of available data

urinary tract infection in which few cases of drug-resistant pathogens were observed (not shown here).

Table 3 shows hazard ratio (HR) and their corresponding 95% CIs for hospital mortality. After adjusting for sex, age, and APACHE II score, significantly higher HR for hospital mortality was found in uses of respirator and central venous catheter, and ICU-acquired infection caused by drug-resistant pathogens, with significantly lower HR for elective and urgent operations and use of urinary catheter. The impact of ICU-acquired infection on hospital mortality was different between drug-sensitive pathogens (HR 1.11, 95% CI: 0.94-1.31) and drug-resistant pathogens (HR 1.42, 95% CI: 1.15-1.77).

Table 3. Factors associated with hospital mortality

	HR	95%CI (lower - upper)	
Sex (vs. Man)	1.06	(0.95 -	1.19)
Age (y.o.)*			
45-54	1.19	(0.94 -	1.49)
55-64	1.06	(0.85 -	1.31)
65-74	1.11	(0.91 -	1.35)
75-	1.33	(1.09 -	1.62)
APACHE II score**			
11-15	1.68	(1.37 -	2.06)
16-20	2.66	(2.18 -	3.25)
21-25	4.28	(3.48 -	5.27)
26-30	5.92	(4.76 -	7.37)
31-	7.88	(6.23 -	9.97)
Operation			
Elective	0.29	(0.24 -	0.34)
Urgent	0.68	(0.59 -	0.77)
Ventilator	1.78	(1.49 -	2.12)
Urinary catheter	0.70	(0.54 -	0.90)
CV catheter	1.23	(1.04 -	1.47)
ICU-acquired infection			
Drug-susceptible	1.11	(0.94 -	1.31)
Drug-resistant	1.42	(1.15 -	1.77)

HR hazard ratio, *CI* confidence interval, * compared to 16–44 y.o., ** compared to 0-10

Severity of Illness and ICU-Acquired Infection

It is still unknown whether severity of illness is related to the development of ICU-acquired infections. When the incidence of ICU-acquired infections is evaluated in terms of severity of illness along with the ICU stay, the incidence of ICU-acquired infections during ICU stays is different according to the severity of illness (Fig. 1). In the most severely ill patients, the incidence of ICU-acquired infections is highest in the early days of ICU admission, while in the least severely ill patients, the incidence of ICU-acquired infections is low in the early days, but increases during the ICU stay up to 20 days. In moderately ill patients, the incidence of ICU-acquired infections does not change markedly during the ICU stay. Therefore, severity affects the incidence ICU-acquired infections; however, this effect on ICU-acquired infections is

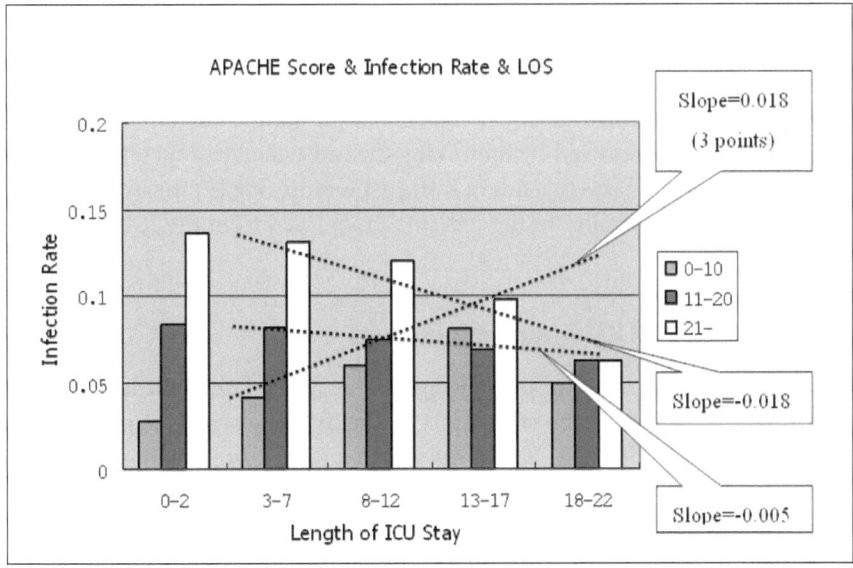

Fig. 1. ICU-acquired infections vs. severity of illness

reversed depending on the severity of illness. In this sense, the general notion that the more severely ill the patients are, the more they develop nosocomial infections cannot be verified.

Performance Measurement of ICUs

Performance of the ICU is usually measured in terms of outcome and process. The incidence of ICU-acquired infection is classified as the process evaluation, while hospital mortality is classified as outcome evaluation. However, the sensitivity of the outcome measurement by hospital mortality is low, because relatively small numbers of the patients die during hospital admission. Additionally, so many confounders are associated with the hospital mortality of ICU patients, including the original disease, severity of illness, development of complications (medical errors and nosocomial infections), patient management (therapeutic, nursing and monitoring capabilities), demographical characteristics (age and gender of the patients), and organisational characteristics (open or closed ICU, staffing). Because the magnitude of contribution of those confounders to mortality is not prioritised, it is extremely difficult to evaluate ICU performance on the individual confounder (risk factor) basis. It is of utmost importance to develop a new statistical model to measure both overall and individual confounder-based performance of the ICU. ICU-acquired infection is one of the most important confounders (risk factors) for the measurement of ICU performance. It is concluded that performance of the ICU is improved by improving the individual risk factors; however, it is extremely difficult to achieve it by just monitoring [9] the overall risk-adjusted hospital mortality of the patients discharged from the ICU.

Strategy for Control ICU-Acquired Infections

The fundamental strategy for preventing ICU-acquired infections is shown in Table 4. The principle of the strategy is 1) clarify the purpose of preventing ICU-acquired infections; 2) standardise the process of infection control; 3) monitor the process and outcome indicators; 4) organise the root cause analysis when outbreak occurs.

Table 4. Strategy for preventing ICU-acquired infections

Purpose of infection control	Improve patient outcome Reduce the cost of medical expenditure
Standardisation of infection control process	Guideline/manual
Process and outcome indicators	Risk-adjusted infection rate Risk-adjusted mortality Risk-adjusted length of stays in ICU and hospital
Outbreak management	Emergency report system Route cause analysis

References

1. Vincent J, Bihari DJ, Suter PM et al (1995) The prevalence of nosocomial infection in intensive care units in Europe. JAMA 274:639–644
2. Kollef MH, Sherman G, Ward S et al (1999) Inadequate antimicrobial treatment of infections: a risk factor for hospital mortality among critically ill patients. Chest 115:462–474
3. Zaidi M, Sifuentes–Osornio J, Rolon AL et al (2002) Inadequate therapy and antibiotic resistance: risk factors for mortality in the intensive care unit. Arch Med Res 33:290–294
4. Alberti C, Brun-Buisson C, Burchardi H (2002) Epidemiology of sepsis and infec-

tion in ICU patients from an international multicentre cohort study. Intensive Care Med 28:108–121

5. Jencks SF, Daley J, Draper D (1988) Interpreting hospital mortality data: the role of clinical risk adjustment. JAMA 260:3611–3616

6. Green J, Wintfeld N, Sharkey P et al (1990) The importance of severity of illness in assessing hospital mortality. JAMA 263:241–246

7. Niederman MS (2001) Impact of antibiotic resistance on clinical outcomes and the cost of care. Crit Care Med 29(suppl):N114–N120

8. Suka M, Yoshida K, Takezawa J (2005) Impact of intensive care unit-acquired infection on hospital mortality in Japan. Environ Health and Prev Med (In press)

9. Yoshida K, Suka M (2004) Report of nosocomial infection in ICU. Annual report of nosocomial infection surveillance. Ministry of Health, Labour and Welfare, Japan

Diagnosis of Pulmonary Embolism

R.G.G. Terzi, M. Mello Moreira

Pulmonary embolism (PE) is a relevant clinical occurrence. Despite advances in diagnostic modalities, PE remains a commonly under diagnosed and lethal disease. In North America it has been reported that the occurrence of 600 000 PE cases are accountable for 50 000 to 200 000 deaths annually [1–4]. Unexpected deaths due to pulmonary embolism are frequently diagnosed post mortem. When diagnosis is established in the emergency department, appropriate anticoagulation is usually effective in reducing the possibility of recurrence and death. Undiagnosed PE has a hospital mortality rate as high as 30% that falls to near 8% if diagnosed and treated properly [3–6]. The mortality rate in ambulatory patients is less than 2% [7]. Clinicians are aware of unexpected deaths due to pulmonary embolism and that appropriate anticoagulation is usually effective in reducing the possibility of recurrence and death. For this reason, image methods are requested whenever there is clinical suspicion of PE. The diagnostic 'gold standard' is pulmonary angiography, against which other imaging modalities have been historically evaluated. Pulmonary angiography is an invasive and expensive procedure, with limited availability and potentially serious complications. There is limited radiological experience with this method as it is not always recognised that, with subsegmental clot, interobserver disagreement occurs in up to one third of cases [8]. Despite being the 'gold standard', pulmonary angiograms are not infallible. A patient with a normal pulmonary angiogram can still expect a 2.2% (95% CI, 0.3 to 8.0%) venous thromboembolic event rate at the one-year follow-up [9].

Over the past two decades the next best investigation has been ventilation-perfusion (V/Q) scintigraphy. When perfusion areas show reduced perfusion not matched by ventilation, the image is suggestive of PE. The mismatched perfusion defect is the diagnostic clue of pulmonary embolism [10]. However, Prospective Investigators of Pulmonary Embolism Diagnosis (PIOPED) investigators reported that PE can only be diagnosed or excluded reliably in a minority of patients by isotope lung scanning [11]. Commonly, a high probability lung scan is considered diagnostic of PE, although the PIOPED investigation showed this is not absolute (some false positives were found in those with previous rather than current PE). When isotope lung scanning is normal, PE is reliably excluded [11, 12]. Follow-up and angiography together suggest that pulmonary embolism occurs among 12% of patients with low-probability scans. Clinical assessment combined with the ventilation/perfusion scan established the diagnosis or exclusion of pulmonary embolism only in a minority of patients—those with clear and concordant clinical and ventilation/perfusion scan findings [11]. However a review of data from all patients with low-probability V/Q scans and a follow-up of six months showed no documentation attributed any deaths to PE. [13]. An indeterminate result is very common in those with symptomatic co-existing cardiopulmonary disease [14] including acute or chronic airways disease and conditions causing intrapulmonary shadowing on the chest radiograph — and in the elderly [15]. Hence, the proposition that further imaging is mandatory in all those with either an indeterminate lung scan or discordant clinical and lung scan probability continues to be emphasised [16]. After an indeterminate ventilation-perfusion study, bilateral leg ultrasound (even in the absence of leg symptoms) may be helpful in showing femoral, popliteal, or calf thrombus. This justifies treatment even when a pulmonary embolus has not been demonstrated [12].

Although a normal perfusion study essentially excludes embolism, it is not so widely valued that, conversely, most patients with pulmonary emboli do not have a high probability result. The PIOPED study reported that of 116 patients with high-probability scans and definitive angiograms, 102 (88%) had pulmonary embolism, but only a minority with pulmonary embolism had high-probability scans (sensitivity, 41%; specificity, 97%) [11]. In subjects investigated for PE, an abnormal chest radiograph increases the prevalence of non-diagnostic scintigrams. A normal pre-test chest radiograph is more often associated with a definitive (normal or high probability) scintigram result [17]. The chest radiograph may be useful in deciding the optimum sequence of investigations. Nevertheless, a reliable classification of the risk of pulmonary embolism is not possible on the basis of non-diagnostic lung scans, regardless of whether the patient has or does not have pulmonary embolism. The interobserver variability is less when the lung scan is evaluated together with the chest X-ray, but even so it is unacceptably high [18]. Present recommendations of the British Thoracic Society regarding isotope lung scanning are that it may be considered as the initial imaging investigation providing that facilities are available on site, *and* a chest radiograph is normal, *and* there is no significant symptomatic concurrent cardiopulmonary disease, *and* standardised reporting criteria are used, *and*, finally, a non-diagnostic result is always followed by further imaging [12]. Such difficulties, together with rather limited availability of nuclear medicine, explains the current interest in spiral computed tomography (spiral CT). Spiral CT angiography is performed during an injection of iodinated contrast medium and can demonstrate emboli directly as filling defects within the pulmonary arteries [19, 20]. Spiral CT is increasingly being used as an adjunct and, more recently, as an alternative to other imaging modalities, and is clearly superior in specificity to ventilation-perfusion isotope scanning [21–26]. There has been a recent trend to analyse the accuracy of spiral CT using clinical outcome measures as opposed to comparison with conventional angiography, and data is accumulating that shows it is safe to withhold anticoagulation when PE is excluded on spiral CT. Early evidence of this came from reports in which it was used in conjunction with other imaging modalities [27, 28]. There has been some concern that spiral CT angiography may miss subsegmental emboli but, given the wide inter-observer variability in reporting subsegmental emboli on pulmonary angiography, this is hard to confirm or refute [29]. Although reports that subsequent pulmonary embolism is low after a negative spiral CT [30], the possibility of recurrent PE and death when the patient is not treated cannot be entirely ruled out. An added advantage of spiral tomography is the fact that, often, causes for chest pain other than pulmonary embolism may be identified [31, 32].

Musset et al. [33] reported a large multicentre study in which all patients were investigated by both spiral CT and leg ultrasound. They studied 1041 consecutive inpatients and outpatients with suspected PE. They left untreated the patients with negative spiral CT and ultrasonography, and who were clinically assessed as having a low or intermediate clinical probability. Those with high clinical probability underwent lung scanning, pulmonary angiography, or both. All patients were followed up for three months and only one of 507 (0.2%) had definite PE. The authors conclude that the withholding of anticoagulant therapy is safe when the clinical probability of PE is assessed as low or intermediate and spiral CT and ultrasonography are negative. Using multi-slice CT technology, Remy-Jardin et al. [34] reported only one recurrence in three months in 91 patients with a negative test who were not anticoagulated. Multi-slice scanners also allow the option of imaging leg veins during the same procedure. Comparison has mainly been made with ultrasound rather than venography and results have been mixed [34–42]. Cham et al. [43] reported that in a group of 541 patients with suspected PE the combined approach identified an additional 18% of patients where only deep venous thrombosis (DVT) could be identified. Disadvantages include an increased radiation dose, particularly to the gonads [44], and longer scanning time. Compared with isotope scanning, spiral CT is quicker to perform, rarely needs to be followed by other imaging and may provide the correct diagnosis when PE has been excluded. According to the recently published British Thoracic Society guidelines for the management of suspected acute PE, spiral CT is now the recommended initial lung imaging modality for non-massive PE. Patients with a good quality negative spiral CT do not require further investigation or treatment for PE [12]. By the same rationale used in indeterminate scintigraphy, computed tomography of the leg veins immediately after spiral CT angiography can identify thrombus [43] without recourse to a separate examination.

Usually lung scans spiral CTs are sufficient to make a definitive diagnosis. Despite undetermined ventilation-perfusion scans, or negative CT, the presence of popliteal or femoral thrombosis in bilateral leg ultrasound or by indirect CT venography justifies anticoagulation.

It has been pointed out that the indiscriminate request of tests to image departments are inducing a large increase in referrals for possible embolus especially in frail, critically ill, elderly people and following recent publicity over the risk of thromboembolism from flying [10]. It is not only the increased workload, which often demands a 24-hour service, but also the costs involved in performing these image exams, often with negative results in a considerable number of patients. In our institution, lung scans and CT angiography proved to be negative in over 40% of the requested exams. The problem is particularly more serious in developing countries where image methods are expensive and usually unavailable. For this reason, non-invasive methods to screen patients for further image tests would reduce the number of patients submitted to lung scans and spiral CTs even in hospitals where these diagnostic facilities are available. Similarly, a positive non-invasive screening test in small community hospitals where definitive diagnostic methods are not available could select the patients that ought to be transferred to larger institutions for further investigation.

Three such screening methods seem promising: 1. clinical pretest assessment; 2. D-dimer assays in blood; 3. volumetric capnography. However, none of these isolated methods have proven infallible in establishing a definitive diagnosis.

Pretest Assessment

The most efficient way to prevent both fatal and non-fatal venous thromboembolism is to use routine prophylaxis for moderate to high risk hospital patients. Despite several recommendations that prophylaxis should be more widely employed, effective prophylaxis is probably insufficient to reduce the incidence of fatal and non-fatal venous thromboembolism. Clinicians should be aware of the risk factors that can lead to DVT and eventually PE. The risk of thromboembolism in a hospital patient depends not only on the illness, trauma, or surgical intervention – which was the reason for admission – but also on pre-existing disease. Age is an important risk factor (Table 1).

Table 1. Thromboembolic risk factors (adapted from [45])

Patient factors	Disease or Surgical Procedure
Age	Trauma
Obesity	Surgery, especially of pelvis, hip, lower limb
Varicose veins	Malignancy, especially pelvic, abdominal, metastatic
Immobility (bed rest for over 4 days)	Heart failure. Recent myocardial infarction
Pregnancy	Paralysis of lower limbs
Puerperium	Infection
High dose estrogen therapy	Inflammatory bowel disease
Previous DVT or PE	Nephrotic syndrome
Thrombophilia	Polycythaemia
Deficiency of antithrombin III, protein C or protein S	Paraproteinemia
Antiphospholipid antibody or lupus anticoagulant	Paroxysmal nocturnal haemoglobinuria
	Bahçet's disease Homocysteinemia

Risk factors have been formatted as predictive scoring systems or simple clinical criteria that indicate safe exclusion of PE. Three of these prediction rules have been published in the last five years.

Good clinical assessment allows better interpretation of isotope scan results. In combination with D-dimer assay (DD), it can substantially reduce the need for imaging. Clinical pretest evaluation in the real world is usually made by junior doctors whose ability to make an accurate estimate of the likelihood of PE is much inferior than that of their seniors [46]. For this reason, a pretest evaluation using defined criteria for assessing clinical probability should result in more uniform accuracy. A simple and effective method of assigning clinical probability was presented by Wells et al. [47]. They collected clinical data on 1239 patients which were analysed by a stepwise logistic regression model. Seven variables were selected to derive a simplified clinical rule. Cut points were identified to classify patients as low (< 2), moderate (2-6), or high (> 6) probability for pulmonary embolism. The method has the advantage of simplicity. The principles introduced successfully for DVT have since shown it to be equally valid and reproducible in PE [48, 49]. It requires that the patient has clinical features compatible with PE – namely, breathlessness and/or tachypnoea, with or without pleuritic chest pain and/or haemoptysis (Table 2).

Table 2. Criteria for assessment of pre-test probability for PE (adapted from [47])

Criteria	Points
Suspected DVT	3.0
An alternative diagnosis is less likely than PE	3.0
Heart rate > 100 beats/min	1.5
Immobilization or surgery in the previous 4 weeks	1.5
Previous DVT or PE	1.5
Hemoptysis	1.0
Malignancy treated < 6 mo	1.0

Score range	Mean probability of PE (%)	Patients with this score (%)	Interpretation of Risk
0-2 points	3.6	40	Low
3-6 points	20.5	53	Moderate
> 6 points	66.7	7	High

Wicki et al. [50] also pooled clinical data involving 986 consecutive patients obtained from the patient history and physical examination. In addition, they included the results of the chest radiograph, electrocardiogram, and arterial blood gas analysis. Again, the seven variables rule was derived by logistic regression. Patients with scores of less than 5 had low pre-test probability of pulmonary embolism, of 5 to 8 had moderate pretest probability, and of greater than 8 had high pretest probability. The prevalence of pulmonary embolism correlated well with pretest probability (Table 3).

Table 3. The seven variables rule for assessment of pre-test probability for PE (adapted from [50])

Criteria	Points
Age 60-79 y	1
Age > 79 y	2
Previous DVT or PE	2
Recent surgery	3
Heart rate > 100 beats/min	1
$PaCO_2 < 36$	2
$PaCO_2$ 36-39	1
$PaO_2 < 49$	4
PaO_2 49-60	3
PaO_2 60-71	2
PaO_2 71-82	1
Chest radiograph – atelectasis	1
Chest radiograph – elevation hemidiaphragm	1

Score range	Mean probability of PE (%)	Patients with this score (%)	Interpretation of Risk
0-4 points	10	49	Low
5-8 points	20.385	44	Moderate
9-12 points	66.781	6	High

Kline et al. [51] reported data on a multicentre, prospective study where the baseline probability of PE in ED patients selected for pulmonary vascular imaging was 19.4%. This study tested the hypothesis that a set of clinical criteria could be developed to define the ED patient with a greater than 40% probability of PE. This model uses two screening variables to assess all patients' age and shock index (heart rate divided by systolic blood pressure). The patient who is either older than 50 years or who has a shock index heartrate/systolic blood pressure (HR/SBP) of more than 1.0, together with any one of four risk factors (unexplained hypoxaemia, unilateral leg swelling, recent history of surgery, or haemoptysis) would have a 42.1% probability of PE (Fig. 1). All of these factors can be determined quickly during a basic history and physical examination, assuming that the ED has a pulse oximeter available. More recently Kline et al. added two more risk factors – previous DVT/PE and oral hormone use [52].

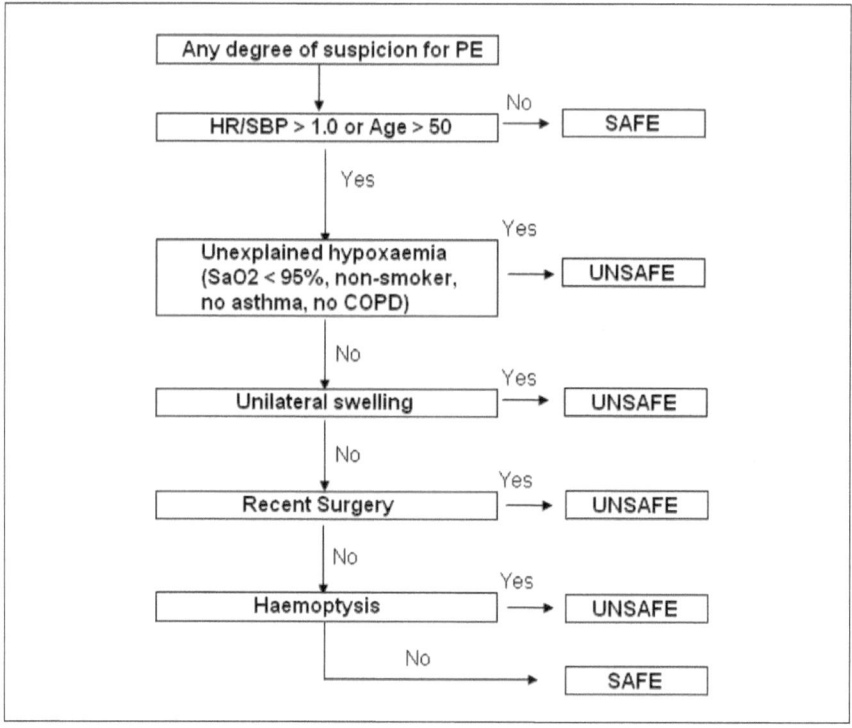

Fig. 1. Decision rule for excluding PE (adapted from [51])

D-Dimer Blood Tests

More than 20 years ago, specific plasma markers for fibrinolysis – D-dimers (DD) – were shown to be increased in patients with thrombosis. However, increased DD do not specify the site of the thrombus. Indeed, DD may be increased in other situations like sepsis, cancer, trauma, renal or cardiac insufficiency, acute coronary ischaemia, pregnancy, and lupus [53–59]. For this reason, specificity varies from 25 to 80% [60]. Bounameaux et al. [61] suggest that costs of image tests may be reduced if DD tests are routinely performed in the Emergency Department in patients with suspected PE. DD are used in several centers for diagnostic PE triage [61–63]. In cases of suspected PE, a negative DD test associated to a low probability lung scan is sufficient enough to exclude PE. However, most tests available to quickly identify abnormal DD in the ED have insufficient sensitivity to exclude PE. Only the ELISA method may reach 100% sensitivity, but it is not a test readily available on a routine basis, for the emergency physician. When available, if an ELISA or Rapid ELISA test proves negative, a suspected PE may be safely excluded.

However, if the test proves positive the diagnosis of PE cannot be established because of the poor specificity – that is, a substantial number of false positives of the test. For this reason, anticoagulation based exclusively on an ELISA DD is not justified. The recent British Thoracic Society guidelines for the management of suspected acute pulmonary embolism advocate that a negative DD test reliably excludes PE in patients with low (SimpliRED, Vidas, MDA) or intermediate (Vidas, MDA) clinical probability and that such patients do not require further imaging tests [12].

Alveolar Dead Space

The third screening tool to rapidly exclude the diagnosis of PE is based on some variables that express the alveolar or physiologic dead space, an objective that has been pursued for several decades. Alveolar dead-space volume occurs in areas of the lung that are ventilated but not perfused, and that contain a very low partial pressure of carbon dioxide (PCO_2). Exhaled dead-space volume dilutes the total amount of carbon dioxide (CO_2) in exhaled breaths relative to the arterial partial pressure of CO_2 ($PaCO_2$). Therefore, the alveolar dead-space volume can be estimated by simultaneously measuring carbon dioxide in exhaled breaths and the $PaCO_2$. Unfortunately, these variables are of limited value because it is difficult to differentiate patients with PE from patients with chronic pulmonary obstructive disease (CPOD), a known pathology that alters the V_A/Q relationship.

Robins et al. [64] reported that the arterial-alveolar carbon dioxide gradient $P(a-et)CO_2$ was over 5 mmHg in seven out of eight patients with proven PE. Subsequently, it has been reported that in one patient with PE, an elevated $P(a-et)CO_2$ effectively was reduced following thrombolysis [65]. Anderson et al. [66] found a sensitivity of 80% and a specificity of 78% when a $P(a-et)CO_2$ of 5 mmHg was used as a cut-off point. However, as an isolated variable the $P(a-et)CO_2$ has limited diagnostic value because chronic obstructive pulmonary disease may develop increased arterial-alveolar PCO_2 gradients.

A second variable, the physiologic dead space (V_D/V_T phys) was employed by Burki [67] to establish that a V_D/V_T phys greater than 0.40 had a sensitivity of 100% and a specificity of 55% to detect PE. However, Eriksson et al. [68] evaluated 38 patients with suspected PE and found that eight out of nine patients with confirmed diagnosis had a V_D/V_T phys over 0.40. They reported that one patient with PE had a V_D/V_T phys of 0.29 and one patient with negative image tests had a V_D/V_T phys of 0.41. Similarly, Anderson et al. [66] reported that only three patients out of five with confirmed PE exhibited a V_D/V_T phys over 0.40 resulting in a sensitivity of 60% and a specificity of 100%.

A third variable, the alveolar dead space (V_D/V_T alv), was evaluated by Kline et al. [69] who reported a sensitivity of 67.2% and a specificity of 76.3%. The alveolar dead space was calculated by subtracting the airway dead space (calculated by the Fowler method) from the physiologic dead space (calculated by the Bohr-Enghoff equation). The cut-off value of the alveolar dead space fraction was set by Kline et al. as 0.20. In view of the finding that the dead-space measurement was normal in almost one third of patients with PE, they emphasised that data does not support the use of the dead space as a sole screening test for PE. Rodger et al. [70] evaluated a fourth variable called steady state ASVDf. This variable is more easily calculated because no physiologic nor anatomic dead space has to be calculated. A simple hand-held capnometer displaying the $PetCO_2$ and an arterial PCO_2 are sufficient to calculate steady state ASVDf. The cut-off value of steady state ASVDf was set by Rodger et al. as 0.15. They reported a sensitivity of 79.5% and a specificity of 70.3%.

The limited value of all these variables lies in the fact that patients with chronic obstructive pulmonary disease (COPD) often have increased V_D/V_T phys due to V_A/Q mismatch. This explains the high incidence of false-positive tests when patients with COPD are tested for suspected PE.

With the objective to refine these tests increasing specificity, Hatle and Rokseth [71] measured the arterial to end tidal carbon dioxide gradient at the end of a long expiration suggesting that a late $P(a\text{-}et)CO_2$ would differentiate PE from COPD. However, this manoeuvre could interfere with steady-state physiology and require the cooperation of a stressed patient in respiratory insufficiency.

To obviate these difficulties, Eriksson et al. [68] described a graphic method to extrapolate $P(a\text{-}et)CO_2$ to a virtual late expiration. They called this variable fDlate. To calculate this variable, $PetCO_2$ is determined at a point on the volumetric capnogram equal to 15% of the total lung capacity (TLC) extending the regression line of Phase III of the volumetric capnogram. Evaluating 38 patients with suspected PE with this method, the cut-off value to differentiate PE from COPD was found to be 0.12 [68]. Further work with fDlate by Olsson et al. [72], who evaluated 233 patients with the same cut-off point showed a sensitivity of 85% and a specificity of 93% including three false negative results. Again, Anderson et al. [66] with the same cut-off point of 0.12 reported a sensitivity of 100% and a specificity of 89% in 12 trauma patients submitted to pulmonary angiography. They reported three false positives cases but no false negative result in their small series.

False positive fDlate results would refer patients for further unnecessary image tests. As a matter of fact, fDlate exhibited a more powerful discrimination between PE and COPD as specificity in these three papers was high. The exclusion of COPD cases resulted in a lower incidence of false fDlate positive results. On the other hand, to date, no large series have reported 100% sensi-

Table 4. Sensitivity and specificity of alveolar dead space derived variables for assessing pretest probability for PE

Test	Reference	Year	Cut-off	Sensitivity	Specificity
P(a-et)CO$_2$	Robins [64]	1959	5mmHg	80.0	78.0
V$_D$ / V$_T$ phys	Burki [67]	1986	0.40	100.0	55.0
fDlate	Eriksson [68]	1989	0.12	85.0	93.0
V$_D$/V$_T$ alv	Kline [69]	2001	0.20	67.2	76.3
ASVDf	Rodger [70]	2001	0.15	79.5	70.3

tivity. False fDlate negative results are not acceptable in this situation because a definitive diagnosis of PE would be missed if further diagnostic work-ups were not carried out. In this case, if no anticoagulation is prescribed, recurrent PE could lead to death.

Recently, Kline et al. [69], Rodger et al. [70], and Johanning et al. [73] have used a new approach to diagnose cases of suspected pulmonary embolism. They combined a dead space derived variable with a fast DD test. From the multicenter Rapid Exclusion of Pulmonary Embolism (REPE) collaborative, pulmonary embolism was diagnosed in 64 subjects and excluded in 316 (16.8% pretest probability of PE). When the requirement of a normal dead-space measurement is added to a normal D-dimer assay, the sensitivity increases from 93.8% to 98.4%. In this study, measured alveolar dead-space fraction functioned well as an adjunctive bedside test when interpreted together with the D-dimer assay. Dead-space measurement did appear to enhance the diagnostic performance of the D-dimer assay [69]. Rodger et al. [70] reported that the combination of a negative D-dimer result and a steady-state end-tidal AVDSf of < 0.15 excluded PE with a sensitivity of 97.8% and a specificity of 38.0%. Johanning [73] et al., evaluating suspected pulmonary embolism, utilised end-tidal CO$_2$ to calculate alveolar space fraction and D-Dimer with a cut-off value of 1000 ng/mL for DD instead of a standard value of 500 ng/mL because they were studying patients admitted to the intensive care unit (ICU). The sensitivity of these combined tests approached 100%. (Table 5).

To the best of our knowledge, there are no published reports combining fDlate with DD. Data from our Institution [74] revealed that in 46 patients with 21 proven PE by lung scans and spiral CTs, sensitivity was 100% and specificity was 80% when both fDlate and DD were negative. Should these preliminary results be confirmed by others, we may see in the near future the emergence of fast and easy ways to exclude PE in the ER, which would avoid almost half of the expensive exams requested today and ease the workload in the Image Departments [10] and reducing overall hospital costs. This may not

Table 5. Sensitivity and specificity of combined alveolar dead space variables and DD for assessing pre-test probability for PE

Alveolar space test	Reference	Sensitivity	Specificity
AVDSf (fraction) + DD	Johanning, 1999 [73]	80.0	100.0
V_D / V_T alv (fraction) + DD	Kline, 2001 [69]	98.4	51.6
AVDSf (fraction) + DD	Rodger, 2001 [70]	97.8	38.0
fDlate (fraction) + DD	Mello, 2004 [74]	100.0	78.0

be so because, as it has been pointed out [75], overuse of DD may have negative consequences. The low specificity leading to a high positive rate of the DD can create the potential for a harmful increase in pulmonary vascular imaging. For this reason, Kline et al. [75] caution that clinicians should pause before ordering a DD test on a patient who is under 50 years of age with a pulse below 100, a pulse oxymetry over 94%, no unilateral leg swelling, no haemoptysis, no history of DVT/PE, no recent surgery and no oral hormone use. Finally, the British Thoracic Society's recent guidelines for the management of suspected acute pulmonary embolism emphasises that blood DD assay should only be considered following assessment of clinical probability. DD assay should not be performed in those with a high clinical probability of PE. Each hospital should provide information on sensitivity and specificity of its DD test [12].

References

1. Anderson FA, Wheeler HB, Goldberg RJ (1991) A population-based perspective of the hospital incidence and case fatality rates of deep venous thrombosis and pulmonary embolism: the Worchester DVT Study. Arch Intern Med 151:933–938
2. Lilienfeld DE, Chan E, Ehland J et al (1990) Mortality from pulmonary embolism in the United States: 1962 to 1984. Chest 98:1067–1072
3. Dalen JE, Alpert JS (1975) Natural history of pulmonary embolism. Prog Cardiovasc Dis 17:257–270
4. Clagett GP, Anderson FA Jr, Heit J et al (1995) Prevention of venous thromboembolism. Chest 108: S312-S334
5. Dismuke SE, Wagner EH (1986) Pulmonary embolism as a cause of death. The changing mortality in hospitalized patients. JAMA 255(15):2039–2042
6. Carson JL, Kelley MA, Duff A et al (1992) The clinical course of pulmonary embolism. N Engl J Med 326:1240–1245
7. Alpert JS, Smith R, Carlson J (1976) Mortality in patients treated for pulmonary embolism. JAMA 236:1477–1480
8. Diffin DC, Leyendecker JR, Johnson SP et al (1998) Effect of anatomic distribution of pulmonary emboli on interobserver agreement in the interpretation of pulmonary angiography. Am J Roentgenol 171:1085

9. Hull RB, Hirsh J, Carter C et al (1993) Pulmonary angiography, ventilation lung scanning, and venography for clinically suspected pulmonary embolism with abnormal perfusion lung scan. Ann Intern Med 98:891–899

10. Dixon AK, Coulden RA, Peters AM (2001) The non-invasive diagnosis of pulmonary embolus. BMJ 323:412–413

11. Anonymous (1990) Value of ventilation/perfusion scan in acute pulmonary embolism. The PIOPED Investigators. JAMA 263:2753–2765

12. Anonymous (2003) British Thoracic Society guidelines for the management of suspected acute pulmonary embolism. British Thoracic Society Standards of Care Committee Pulmonary Embolism Guideline Development Group. Thorax 58:470–483

13. Rajendran JG, Jacobson AF (1999) Review of 6-month mortality following low-probability lung scans. Arch Intern Med 159:349–352

14. Hartmann I, Hagen P, Melissant C et al (2000) Diagnosing acute pulmonary embolism: effect of chronic obstructive pulmonary disease on the performance of D-dimer testing, ventilation/perfusion scintigraphy, spiral computed tomographic angiography, and conventional angiography. Am J Respir Crit Care Med 162:2232–2237

15. Righini M, Goehring C, Bounameaux H et al (2000) Effects of age on the performance of common diagnostic tests for pulmonary embolism. Am J Med 109:357–361

16. Worsley DF, Alavi A (2001) Radionuclide imaging of acute pulmonary embolism. Radiol Clin N Am 39:1035–1052

17. Forbes KP, Reid JH, Murchison JT (2001) Do preliminary chest X-ray findings define the optimum role of pulmonary scintigraphy in suspected pulmonary embolism? Clin Radiol 56:397–400

18. Broekhuizen-de Gast HS, Tiel-van Buul MM, Ubbink M et al (2000) The value of the 'non-diagnostic' lung scan - further classification as to the risk of pulmonary embolism is not reliable. Ned Tijdschr Geneeskd 144:1537–1542

19. Remy-Jardin M, Remy J, Wattinne L et al (1992) Central pulmonary thromboembolism: diagnosis with spiral volumetric CT with the single-breath-hold technique: comparison with pulmonary angiography. Radiology 185:381–387

20. Goodman LR, Lipchik RJ, Kuzo RS (1997) Acute pulmonary embolism: the role of computed tomographic imaging. J Thorac Imaging 12:83–86

21. Hartmann I, Hagen P, Melissant C et al (2000) Diagnosing acute pulmonary embolism: effect of chronic obstructive pulmonary disease on the performance of D-dimer testing, ventilation/perfusion scintigraphy, spiral computed tomographic angiography, and conventional angiography. Am J Respir Crit Care Med 162:2232–2237

22. Mayo JR, Remy-Jardin M, Muller NL et al (1997) Pulmonary embolism: prospective comparison of spiral CT with ventilation-perfusion scintigraphy. Radiology 205:447–452

23. Garg K, Welsh CH, Feyerabend AJ et al (1998) Pulmonary embolism: diagnosis with spiral CT and ventilation-perfusion scanning - correlation with pulmonary angiographic results or clinical outcome. Radiology 208:201–208

24. Van Rossum AB, Pattynama PM, Mallens WM et al (1998) Can helical CT replace scintigraphy in the diagnostic process in suspected pulmonary embolism? A retrolective-prolective cohort study focusing on total diagnostic yield. Eur Radiol 8:90–96

25. Blachere H, Latrabe V, Montaudon M et al (2000) Pulmonary embolism revealed on

helical CT angiography: comparison with ventilation-perfusion radionuclide lung scanning. Am J Roentgenol 174:1041–1047

26. Cueto SM, Cavanaugh SH, Benenson RS et al (2001) Computed tomography scan versus ventilation-perfusion lung scan in the detection of pulmonary embolism. J Emerg Med 21:155–164

27. Ferretti GR, Bosson JL, Buffaz PD et al (1997) Acute pulmonary embolism: role of helical CT in 164 patients with intermediate probability at ventilation-perfusion scintigraphy and normal results at duplex US of the legs. Radiology 205:453–458

28. Lorut C, Ghossains M, Horellou M et al (2000) A non-invasive diagnostic strategy including spiral computed tomography in patients with suspected pulmonary embolism. Am J Respir Crit Care Med 162:1413–1418

29. Stein PD, Henry JW, Gottschalk A (1999) Reassessment of pulmonary angiography for the diagnosis of pulmonary embolism: relation of interpreter agreement to the order of the involved pulmonary arterial branch. Radiology 210:689–691

30. Cooper TJ, Protero DL, Gillett MG et al (1992) Laboratory investigations in the diagnosis of pulmonary thromboembolism. Quart J Med 301:369–376

31. Coche EE, Muller NL, Kim KI (1998) Acute pulmonary embolism: ancillary findings at spiral CT. Radiology 207:753–760

32. Cross JJL, Kemp PM, Walsh CG et al (1998) A randomized trial of spiral CT and ventilation perfusion scintigraphy for the diagnosis of pulmonary embolism. Clin Radiol 53:177–182

33. Musset D, Parent F, Meyer G et al (2002) Diagnostic strategy for patients with suspected pulmonary embolism: a prospective multicentre outcome study. Lancet 360:1914–1920

34. Remy-Jardin M, Tillie-Leblond I, Szapiro D et al (2002) CT angiography of pulmonary embolism in patients with underlying respiratory disease: impact of multislice CT (MSCT) on image quality and negative predictive value. Eur Radiol 12:1971–1978

35. Cham MD, Yankelevitz DF, Shaham D et al (2000) Deep venous thrombosis: detection by using indirect CT venography. The Pulmonary Angiography-Indirect CT Venography Cooperative Group. Radiology 216:744–751

36. Duwe K, Shiau M, Budorick N et al (2000) Evaluation of the lower extremity veins in patients with suspected pulmonary embolism: a retrospective comparison of helical CT venography and sonography. Am J Roentgenol 175:1525–1531

37. Garg K, Kemp JL, Wojcik D et al (2000) Thromboembolic disease: comparison of combined CT pulmonary angiography and venography with bilateral leg sonography in 70 patients. Am J Roentgenol 175:997–1001

38. Ghaye B, Szapiro D, Willems V et al (2000) Combined CT venography of the lower limbs and spiral CT angiography of pulmonary arteries in acute pulmonary embolism: preliminary results of a prospective study. J Belg Radiol 83:271–278

39. Au VW, Walsh G, Fon G (2001) Computed tomography pulmonary angiography with pelvic venography in the evaluation of thrombo-embolic disease. Australas Radiol 45:141–145

40. Loud PA, Katz DS, Bruce DA et al (2001) Deep venous thrombosis with suspected pulmonary embolism: detection with combined CT venography and pulmonary angiography. Radiology 219:498–502

41. Nicolas M, Debelle L, Laurent V et al (2001) Incremental lower extremity CT venography, a simplified approach for the diagnosis of deep venous thrombosis in patients with pulmonary embolism. J Radiol 82:251–256

42. Peterson DA, Kazerooni EA, Wakefield TW et al (2001) Computed tomographic

venography is specific but not sensitive for diagnosis of acute lower-extremity deep venous thrombosis in patients with suspected pulmonary embolus. J Vasc Surg 34:798–804

43. Cham MD, Yankelevitz DF, Shaham D et al (2000) Deep venous thrombosis: detection by using indirect CT venography. The Pulmonary Angiography-Indirect CT Venography Cooperative Group. Radiology 216:744–751

44. Rademaker J, Griesshaber V, Hidajat N et al (2001) Combined CT pulmonary angiography and venography for diagnosis of pulmonary embolism and deep vein thrombosis: radiation dose. J Thorac Imaging 16:297–299

45. Anonymous (1992) Risk of and prophylaxis for venous thromboembolism in hospital patients. Thromboembolic Risk Factors (THRIFT) Consensus Group. BMJ 305:567–574

46. Rosen M, Sands D, Morris J et al (2000) Does a physician's ability to accurately assess the likelihood of pulmonary embolism increase with training? Acad Med 75:1199–1205

47. Wells PS, Anderson DR, Rodger M et al (2000) Derivation of a simple clinical model to categorize patients probability of pulmonary embolism: increasing the models utility with the SimpliRED D-dimer. Thromb Haemost 83:416–420

48. Wells PS, Ginsberg JS, Anderson DR et al (1998) Use of a clinical model for safe management of patients with suspected pulmonary embolism. Ann Intern Med 129:997–1005

49. Wells PS, Anderson DR, Rodger M et al (2001) Excluding pulmonary embolism at the bedside without diagnostic imaging: management of patients with suspected pulmonary embolism presenting to the emergency department by using a simple clinical model and D-dimer. Ann Intern Med 135:98–107

50. Wicki J, Perneger TV, Junod AF et al (2001) Assessing clinical probability of pulmonary embolism in the emergency ward. Arch Intern Med. 161:92–97

51. Kline JA, Nelson RD, Jackson RE et al (2002) Criteria for the safe use of D-dimer testing in emergency department patients with suspected pulmonary embolism: a multicenter US study. Ann Emerg Med. 39:144–152

52. Kline JA, Mitchell AM, Kabrhel C et al (2004) Clinical criteria to prevent unnecessary diagnostic testing in emergency department patients with suspected pulmonary embolism. J Thromb Haemost. Aug 2(8):1247–55

53. Hager K, Platt D (1995) Fibrin degeneration product concentration (D-dimers) in the course of ageing. Gerontology 41:159–165

54. Kruskal JB, Commerford PJ, Franks JJ et al (1987) Fibrin and fibrinogen related antigens in patients with stable and unstable coronary disease. N Eng J Med 317:1362–1365

55. Gustafsson C, Blomback M, Britton M (1990) Coagulation factors and the increased risk of stroke in non valvular atrial fibrillation. Stroke 21:47–51

56. Becker DM, Philbrick JT, Bachhuber TL et al (1996) D-dimer tesing and acute venous thromboembolism. Arch Intern Med 156:939–946

57. Giroud M, Dutrillaux F, Lemesle M et al (1998) Coagulation abnormalities in lacunar and cortical ischaemic stroke are quite different. Neurol Res 20:15–18

58. Foti M, V Gurewich (1980) Fibrin degradation products and impedance plethysmography. Arch Intern Med 140:903–906

59. Whitaker A, Rowe E, Masci P et al (1980) Identification of D dimer-E complex in disseminated intravascular coagulation. Thromb Res 18:453–459

60. Kelly J, Rudd A, Lewis RR et al (2002) Plasma D-Dimers in the diagnosis of venous thromboembolism. Arch Intern Med 162:747–56

61. Bounameaux H, Schneider PA, Reber G et al (1989) Measurement of plasma D-dimer for diagnosisof deep vein thrombosis. Am J Cl Pathol 91:82–85

62. Bounameaux H, P de Moerloose, A Perrier et al (1994) Plasma measurement of D-dimer as diagnosis aid in suspected venous thromboembolism: an overview. Thromb Haemost 71:1–6

63. Lorut C, JP Laaban, A Achkar et al (1996) Diagnostic value of plasma D-dimer in suspected venous thromboembolism. Sem Hôp Paris 72:673–685

64. Robins ED, Julian DG, Travis DM et al (1959) A physiologic approach to the diagnosis of acute pulmonary embolism. New Engl J Med. 260:586–591

65. Thys F, ElamLy A, Marion E, Roesler J et al (2001) PaCO2/ETCO2 gradient: early indicator of thrombolysis efficacy in a massive pulmonary embolism. Resuscitation 49:105–108

66. Anderson JT, Owings JT, Goodnight JE (1999) Bedside non invasive detection acute pulmonary embolism in critically ill surgical patients. Archives of Surgery 134:869–875

67. Burki N (1986) The dead space to tidal volume ratio in the diagnosis of pulmonary embolism. Am Rev Respir Dis 133:679–685

68. Eriksson L, Wollmer P, Olsson CG et al (1989) Diagnosis of pulmonary embolism based upon alveolar deadspace analysis. Chest 96:357–362

69. Kline JA, Israel EG, Michelson EA et al (2001) Diagnostic accuracy of bedside D-dimer assay and alveolar dead-space measurement for rapid exclusion of pulmonary embolism. JAMA 285:761–768

70. Rodger MA, Jones G, Rasuli P et al (2001) Steady-state end-tidal alveolar dead space fraction and D-dimer. Chest 120:115–119

71. Hatle L, Rokseth R (1974) The arterial to end-expiratory carbon dioxide tension gradient in acute pulmonary embolism and other cardiopulmonary diseases. Chest 66:352–357

72. Olsson K, Jonson B, Olsson CG et al (1998) Diagnosis of pulmonary embolism by measurement of alveolar dead space. J Int Med 244:199–207

73. Johanning JM, Veverka TJ, Bays RA et al (1999) Evaluation of suspected pulmonary embolism utilizing end-tidal CO2 and D-Dimer. Am J Surg 178:98–102

74. Moreira MM, Terzi RGG (2005) Triagem não invasiva para a exclusão diagnóstica de pacientes com suspeita de tromboembolismo pulmonar (TEP). Revista Brasileira de Terapia Intensiva 16:124–137

75. Kline JA, Wells PS (2003) Methodology for a rapid protocol to rule out pulmonary embolism in the emergency department. Ann Emerg Med 42:266–275

Critical Care Nursing, a WorldWide Perspective

G. WILLIAMS

Introduction

In October 2001, at the 8th World Congress of Intensive Care and Critical Care Medicine in Sydney, Australia, a meeting was held in one of the conference halls. Present were about 70 critical care nurses from 15 countries who had gathered to discuss the benefits of an international network of critical care nurses either through their representative national associations or as individuals.

Presentations followed from members of the European Federation of Critical Care Nursing Associations (EfCCNa), an organisation that had formed two years earlier. A presentation from Belle Rogado of the Philippines summarised the developments of critical care nursing in Asia. Ged Williams from Australia presented the results of his survey of critical care nursing organisations and their members from 24 different countries [1]. Others in the audience expressed their own perspectives on critical care nursing in many different countries around the world.

By the end of the four-hour meeting, a draft constitution had been created and approved by the group (Table 1). The World Federation of Critical Care Nurses (WFCCN) was born! Eight national associations of critical care nurses had agreed to join together to establish the first Council of the WFCCN and had provided representatives to manage the Council. In addition, four of the new council members were nominated and elected by the audience to form the inaugural core administration – Chair, Secretary, Treasurer, and Trade Liaison.

Background

Critical care nursing is most strongly associated with intensive care nursing. Intensive care units (ICUs) emerged in North America and parts of Europe in the late 1950s and were most commonly associated with ventilation of

Table 1. WFCCN Constitution: Philosophy, Purpose, and Objectives (only)

Philosophy:
    The philosophy of the WFCCN is to assist critical care nursing associations and nurses regardless of age, gender, nation, colour, religious beliefs, or social background in the pursuit of the objectives of the WFCCN.

Purpose:
    The purpose of the WFCCN is to link critical care nursing associations with nurses throughout the world, to strengthen the influence and contribution of critical care nurses to health care globally, and to be a collective voice and advocate for critical care nurses and patients at an international level.

Objectives:
    (1) To represent critical care nurses and critical care nursing at an international level.
    (2) To improve the standard of care provided to critically ill patients and their families throughout the countries of the world.
    (3) To advance the art and science of critical care nursing in all countries throughout the world.
    (4) To promote cooperation, collaboration, and support for critical care nursing organisations, and individuals.
    (5) To improve the recognition given to critical care nursing throughout the world.
    (6) To maintain and improve effective cooperation between all health professionals, institutions, agencies, and charities who have a professional interest in the care of critically ill patients.
    (7) To establish standards for education, practice, and management of critical care nursing.
    (8) To foster and support research initiatives that advance critical care nursing and patient/family care.
    (9) To encourage and enhance education programs in critical care nursing throughout the world.
    (10) To provide conferences, written information, and continuing education for critical care nurses.

patients suffering from the poliomyelitis epidemics of the era [2]. Further developments in medicine and nursing led to the establishment of ICUs in many parts of the affluent world and further expansion of these units led to improvements in the knowledge and ability to save more lives. By the late 1960s, intensive care medicine was beginning to define itself as a new specialty and some doctors decided to build a career in this very dynamic and exciting field. Of course, medical intervention is impossible without nursing support, and so nurses wishing to specialise in this field emerged concurrently [2].

In 1972, the first World Congress of Intensive Care and Critical Care Medicine was held in London, and whilst the focus was on the sharing of new practices and treatments among intensive care doctors, the participants at the conference numbered many nurses from many parts of the world also. Future meetings of the World Congress of Intensive Care and Critical Care Medicine would see collectives of critical care nurses meet to discuss a possible worldwide organisation of critical care nurses that would take almost two decades to be realised (Table 2).

With further developments, intensive care itself became more sophisticated and with each new development came sub-specialties of intensive care. Sub-specialties of intensive care are more broadly defined collectively as 'critical care' and may include coronary care, cardiothoracic ICU, neuroscience, medical ICU, surgical ICU, paediatric, neonatal, transplantation, recovery, and trauma to name a few.

Different forms of collaboration have emerged among critical care nurses in different countries. Critical care nursing special interest groups have either formed within generic national nursing associations or they have emerged as associate members of intensive care medicine societies. In many countries such models still exist. As they develop professionally, some critical care nursing groups have formed their own unique entity as critical care nursing asso-

Table 2. History of formal International Dialogue aimed at forming stronger international networks between critical care nurses and CCNOs

1985	4th World Congress - Tel Aviv – Australian Critical Care Nurses first ask to be admitted to WFSICCM
1989	5th World Congress - Kyoto - Australia and USA applications accepted by WFSICCM. Sarah Sandford (USA) and Lorraine Ferguson (Australia) ask for nursing position on the board
1993	6th World Congress - Madrid - CCNOs from Australia, USA, Britain and Spain formally admitted to WFSICCM and Nursing member appointed to board (Belinda Atkinson, England). Madrid Declaration on the Preparation of Critical Care Nurses announced and signed. CCNOs pledge to improve international communication, collaboration, and expansion
1994	AACN Global Connections Conference, Toronto – CCNOs meet during this conference, share visions and pledge to improve international communication, collaboration, and expansion
1997	7th World Congress – Ottawa – CCNOs meet during this conference, share visions, and pledge to improve international communication, collaboration, and expansion
2000	BACCN - Global Connections Conference, Edinburgh – Ged Williams presents results of the world CCNOs survey and outlines possibilities for a World Federation of Critical Care Nursing Organisations

AACN American Association of Critical Care Nurses, BACCN British Association of Critical Care Nurses, CCNO Critical Care Nursing Organisation, WFSICCM World Federation of Intensive Care and Critical Care Medicine

ciations, although strong links to their medical colleagues or the national generic nursing association usually remain in tact long after the separation.

Methodology

The worldwide study of critical care nursing organisations and their activities [1] sought to find out how many such organisations of critical care nurses existed in the world. At the time of the study many limitations existed: Email was a relatively new tool and one not possessed by many nurses, especially in developing countries; the WFSICCM was medically focused and access to nurse representatives through the member societies of WFSICCM was often difficult; and the International Council of Nurses, whilst helpful itself, found it difficult to access critical care specific nursing associations in member countries. In order to find critical care nursing representatives, word of mouth and loose networks of individuals were by far the most successful forms of finding and communicating with key persons who wanted to help with the original study. Eventually, a representative sample of critical care nursing associations (and/or individual critical care nurses in countries without critical care nursing associations) was identified to help inform people of the key issues and activities of critical care nurses in those countries represented in the study.

Surveys were distributed to 44 individuals/countries by email, fax, and post over a twelve-month period (1999–2000) to try and capture as many diverse perspectives as possible. All surveys were written in English (another limiting factor in the study).

Results

Twenty-four surveys were completed and returned (Table 3).

Issues important to critical care nurses around the world: When asked to identify the issues that were currently important to them, almost every country identified inadequate staffing levels as being the most important issue for critical care nurses (Table 4). Other important issues included working conditions, access to quality educational programs, and wages.

Services and supports provided by critical care nursing organisations to their members: The respondents said professional representation, national conferences, and standards for educational courses were the three most important activities provided for critical care nurses by their national association. Interestingly, the provision of research-funding grants, a website and

Table 3. Countries responding to survey (number of members in society). Phase II

Americas	Europe		Asia & South Pacific
Canada (1200)	Iceland(75)	Slovenia(300)	Korea(2000)
USA (65 000)	Britain(3200)	Greece (115)	Hong Kong(500)
Mexico (200)	Norway (1700)	Germany(850)	Australia (2500)
	Belgium (450)	Denmark (2700)	Taiwan (N/A)
	Italy (2500)	Ireland(400)	New Zealand(130)
	Finland (1456)	France (225)	Japan (1300)
			India (N/A)
			Turkey (300)
			Philippines (350)

industrial/union representation were ranked very low compared with the other options in this question (Table 5).

Participation in an International Society (Network) of Critical Care Nursing Organisations (CCNOs): All but two countries responded positively to this suggestion. The remaining two stated that they did not know and would need to discuss the issue further. Respondents identified several activities they thought such an international society could provide. These activities were then grouped into the categories of practice, education, research, and

Table 4. Mean Responses for important Issues for Critical Care Nurses

[a]Issue	World (Mean)
Staffing levels	9.24
Working conditions	8.86
Access to quality educational programs	8.76
Wages	8.52
Formal practice guidelines/competences	8.38
Work activities/roles	8.33
Teamwork	8.29
Extended/advanced practice	7.90
Relationships with doctors	7.76
Formal credentialling processes	7.60
Use of technologies	7.38
Facilities and equipment	7.24
Relationships with other nursing orgs	6.90
Relationship with other health groups	6.76

[a]scale: 1 = not important; 10 = very important)

Table 5. Services/activities provided by Critical Care National Organisation and importance attached to each service/activity

[a]Service or Activity	Provided	World (Mean)
Professional representation	17 (71%)	8.75
National Conferences	19 (79%)	8.67
Standards for educational courses	13 (54%)	8.67
Practice standards/guidelines	16 (67%)	8.40
Workshops/Education forums	18 (75%)	8.29
Credentialling process	12 (50%)	8.25
Journal	16 (67%)	7.93
Local Conferences	17 (71%)	7.81
Newsletter	16 (67%)	7.73
Initiate, conduct or lead research studies	13 (54%)	7.58
Training/Skill acquisition course (e.g. Advanced life support)	13 (54%)	7.42
Study/education grants	9 (38%)	7.00
Industrial/union representation	6 (25%)	7.20
Website	15 (63%)	6.79
Research grants	7 (29%)	6.43

[a]scale: 1 = not important; 10 = very important)

professional. Practice activities included exchange of information, staff exchange programs, and bench-marking practices. Educational activities encompassed study tours and sharing educational programs and ideas. The research-related activity named was facilitating the conduct of international research. Professional activities comprised the bulk of the suggestions, and included gaining access to conference speakers, worldwide conferences, and the development of international standards that would inform practice.

When asked what activities and services an international society of CCNOs might offer member associations and critical care nurses internationally, most respondents suggested that a website, international conferences, and study exchanges would be of most value, while the provision of international education, research support, and a journal were also seen as being of value (Table 6).

Nineteen of the 24 respondents suggested English should be the first language of choice for international communication. When asked the extent to which they could financially contribute to the administration and communication functions of an international society, one country responded that no support could be provided and eight did not know. Only 15 indicated that they could provide up to $200 (US) per annum in financial support, while seven indicated they could provide in excess of $750 (US) per annum.

Table 6. Importance of potential services/activities for an International Society of CCNOs

[a]Service and Activity	World (Mean)
Website	9.19
Coordinate/Support in international conference	8.90
Coordinate/Support international study exchanges	8.86
Provide international guidelines/principles relevant to critical care practice	8.74
Coordinate/Support international education	8.67
Coordinate/Support international research projects	8.57
Journal	8.52
Make representation to national and international bodies on issues of health, human-society	8.43
Newsletter	7.48

[a]scale: 1 = not important; 10 = very important

Discussion

Establishing the World Federation of Critical Care Nurses

As mentioned in the introduction, the WFCCN had only eight original member countries and no money! The first Council met the day after inauguration to set a plan for the future. A very important and strategic step was to invite the newly elected President of WFSICCM, Dr Philip Lumb, to the meeting. His words were prophetic and inspiring to the group, as he articulated his desire that WFCCN and WFSICCM maintain close and cooperative linkages during this period of change and development. Dr Lumb expressed regret that the number of critical care nursing societies in WFSICCM had dwindled, but acknowledged that many of the medical societies contained nursing members and that WFSICCM would retain a non-physician member on its Council. This person (Ged Williams) would be a conduit for communication between the two World Federations.

The immediate goals of the WFCCN were set out at this meeting; they are:

- To promote the existence of the WFCCN to potential member associations and encourage application and membership
- To create an official journal of the WFCCN to be distributed to all member associations and their members
- To develop a website containing relevant information that is easily accessible to critical care nurses the world over
- To explore long-term legal, financial, and constitutional arrangements that will best serve the purposes and objectives of the WFCCN and its member associations

Achievements of the WFCCN (As of 2005)

In less than four years the WFCCN has achieved the following:
* Twenty-five member organisations (Table 7)
* Three corporate sponsors: CodeBlue Nursing Agency (Australia), Abbot Laboratories/Hospira, and Datex Ohmeda
* Establishment of a website: www.wfccn.org
* Establishment of an online journal, *CONNECT The World of Critical Care Nursing:* www.wfccn.org/Pages/journal

Table 7. Members of WFCCN as at June 2005-06-27

Core Administration:

> Chairman - Ged Williams (Australia)
> Secretary - Ma. Isabelita C. Rogado (Phillipines)
> Treasurer - Bernice Budz (Canada)
> Trade & Sponsor Representative - Gerardo Jasso Ortega (Mexico)

Members

> Argentina – Laura Alberto
> Brazil – Denis Moura Jr
> Chile - Celia Ortiz
> China - Liu Shuyuan
> Cyprus - Evanthia Georgiou
> Denmark - Birte Baktoft
> Hong Kong - Esther Wong
> Iceland - Rosa Thorsteinsdottir
> Japan - Satoki Ito
> Netherlands - Wouter. de Graaf
> New Zealand - Gordon Speed
> Norway - Lisbet Grenager
> Slovenia - Slavica Klancar
> Spain - Jeronimo Romero-Nieva Lozano
> South Africa - Shelley Schmollgruber
> South Korea - Dong Oak Debbie Kim
> Sweden - Monica Magnusson
> Taiwan - Yolanda Huang
> United Kingdom - John Albarran
> United States of America - Wendy Berke

To be confirmed:

> Singapore
> Turkey

- Annual national conference run in conjunction with member or affiliate societies – 2004 (Cambridge UK, with BACCN), 2005 (Argentina with WFSICCM), 2006 (Manila, Philippines with CCNAPI)
- Admission to the International Council of Nursing and official participation in the 23rd Quadrennial meeting of ICN in Taiwan, May 2005
- Development of two key Position Statements:
- Provision of Critical Care Nursing Education
- Provision of Critical Care Nursing Workforce
- Strategic linkages and support to the emergence and growth of regional critical care nursing federations in: Europe (EfCCNa), Asia-Pacific (APFC-CN), and South America (currently under discussion and development)
- Ongoing and healthy relationship with WFSICCM – Joint meeting of both Councils to occur 30 August 2005
- World-wide study of critical care nursing in progress – expected publication in 2006. This study is similar to that discussed earlier [1]

Creating a Sustainable Future for Critical Care Nursing WorldWide

From humble beginnings, the world of critical care nurses and the WFCCN are demonstrating the capacity to communicate effectively across various language, cultural, and geographical barriers; to get organised; and to generate resources to support mutually agreed activities and goals. The WFCCN provides a legitimate forum for the expression of a collective opinion of what the world of critical care nurses believes to be important issues and activities to improve the effectiveness of critical care nursing. Furthermore, and more importantly, the WFCCN is an advocacy body for representing the needs of critically ill patients and their families – arguably some of the most vulnerable people in our communities. This role and responsibility cannot be managed alone for it is too great for one group to shoulder.

The WFCCN recognises the important base from which it's supported and the important strategic advantages of working collaboratively with those groups who share a similar philosophy and mission. Its roots stem from well-educated but pragmatic clinical nurses who provide 24-hour a day, seven-day-a-week care to the critical ill in every part of the world. These nurses meet and discuss issues, ideas, and solutions, they get organised in their hospitals and share these ideas with their jurisdictional and national organisations. The national organisations of critical care nurses contain sophisticated and politically astute leaders who work with other national bodies and governments to analyse the issues presented to them, to mobilise resources and action, and to address the concerns and ultimately improve the quality of care afforded the critically ill. At an international level, the WFCCN brings together the collective issues, where the ideas and experiences of its member associations can be shared across geographic, cultural, and political boundaries so that nurses can learn from one another, help one another, and ensure that the care of their patients is forever improving. Furthermore, WFCCN establishes strategic alliance with WFSICCM, ICN, the World Health Organisation, and others over time to ensure the needs of critical care nurses, patients, and their families are acknowledged in the appropriate policy making forums of the world.

Over time, the WFCCN will research and develop more information on issues of collective importance – position statements addressing education and workforce requirements were two very obvious and pressing issues addressed in the first instance. It is foreseeable that in the next four to five years, research into clinical and humanitarian issues will emerge as priorities. Linking stronger member societies to emerging societies in developing countries will see the strengthening and equalization of standards of care internationally. Sharing of knowledge, ideas, and resources (financial, intellectual, and human) at an international level, no matter how meagre to start with, will create a culture of goodwill and ultimate improvement in our specialty.

This is a utopian end to an otherwise pragmatic and tough reality. The formative years of the WFCCN have been quiet but notable; the path is now laid for a more productive and effective future.

References

1. Williams G, Chaboyer W, Thorsteinsdottir R et al (2001) World Wide Overview of Critical Care Nursing Organisations and their Activities. International Nursing Review 48:208–217
2. Wiles V, Daffurn K (2002) There's a bird in my hand and a bear by my bed – I must be in ICU: the pivotal years of Australia critical care nursing. Australian College of Critical Care Nurses, Carlton, Australia

Cost of Care in Critical Illness

T.A. WILLIAMS, G.J. DOBB

Intensive care units (ICUs) are an expensive [1–4] and growing [4, 5] part of health care in developed nations. Greater consumer expectations, ageing populations [6, 7], demand for sophisticated technologies [8], and, in the United States (US), defensive medicine [9] are increasing demand for intensive care. Intensive care is increasingly being provided to older and sicker patients, many of whom would not have been referred for intensive care in the past [10]. The proportion of health care resources needed may be seen as disproportionate [2, 11–23] but intensive care requires many highly skilled staff in a complex, expensive, technology-driven environment [4].

Costing studies in ICUs provide information about the costs incurred in the unit, and how these relate to therapeutic activity, patient characteristics, and patient outcomes [24]. Analysing patient-specific ICU costs to identify cost drivers may improve use of ICU resources [24–26]. However, there is little information on the overall cost-effectiveness of intensive care [27, 28]. Also, the treatment needed by intensive care patients varies considerably in type, duration and cost, making it extremely difficult to predict patient resource use. Few studies measure actual costs. Average daily costs are usually calculated and these do not reflect the variation in resource use between individual patients [29].

Health Economics

Evaluation of the costs and benefits of ICU requires some understanding of health economics. Health economics is concerned with determining the best way of using available healthcare resources to maximise the health of the community [30]. Because health care resources are scarce, choices must be made about how the available resources should be shared. The benefits of a particular choice should exceed the benefits of any alternative not chosen to ensure that the best possible outcomes are obtained for a given level of expenditure [31].

Techniques

Clinical costing (bottom-up) captures costs at the point of service delivery [32]. The large amount of data collected and sophisticated costing information systems used are very demanding [32]. Cost modelling (top-down approach) starts with the total costs of a service's operations and distributes costs through patient care cost centres to a case-mix category to produce an estimated cost for specific diagnosis related groups [32].

Economic analyses measure and value the resource consumption or costs in relation to the outcomes they produce [30]. Data for economic analysis of healthcare programmes or interventions may be collected prospectively during a randomised trial to assess the relative efficacy of alternative treatments. However, they may not reflect 'real' practice and the duration of trials may truncate the period over which costs and benefits accrue [30]. Economic analysis may also use estimates of cost and outcomes from a variety of primary sources such as administrative databases.

Economic evaluations systematically consider all possible costs and their consequences to determine the best use of available healthcare resources. Although they do not form the sole basis for decision-making, economic evaluations offer useful information at different levels of decision-making [30]. Although the process of measuring costs is similar in all kinds of economic evaluations, the clinical outcome measured determines the type of economic evaluation [30]. Economic evaluations that consider only one programme or deal with cost only or consequences only (but not both) are considered partial economic evaluations. Both costs and effects depend on the perspective chosen for the economic evaluation. Economic evaluation may be classified as a cost-minimisation analysis, cost-effectiveness analysis, cost-utility analysis, or cost-benefit analysis.

Cost-Minimisation Analysis

In cost-minimisation analysis, the outcomes are equivalent regardless of the units used to measure them. In the other types of economic analyses, the outcomes are evaluated in natural units such as years of life saved (cost-effectiveness analysis), a non-monetary index such as quality-adjusted life-years (QALYs) or healthy year equivalents (cost-utility analysis), or dollars (cost-benefit analysis) [33].

Cost-Effectiveness Analysis

Cost-effectiveness analyses compare the costs and consequences of various programmes or interventions that have a common effect (such as life-years saved), assuming that the outcome of interest is worthwhile and clinically relevant. They make no attempt to measure the value placed by the decision-makers (e.g., patients, healthcare providers, society, etc.) on that outcome. However, reporting only a single, summary measure (such as life-years saved), other competing or concurrent health outcomes, such as quality of life of the survivor, the adverse effects of the intervention, or other measures of morbidity are ignored [30]. Using life-years saved as an outcome tends to favour conditions or interventions that affect survival and discriminate against chronic diseases that have little effect on mortality but influence morbidity, especially in the elderly, who have fewer years available to be saved [30].

Cost-Utility Analysis

Cost-utility analysis acknowledges the multidimensional nature of health outcomes by incorporating morbidity and mortality effects into a single, non-monetary summary measurement. Different interventions can then be compared for their effect on both duration and quality of life and at different levels of effect. The Quality Adjusted Life Year (QALY) is a health status measure in which each definable health status is assigned a weight from 0 (for death) to 1 (for full health). The time spent in each health state is then multiplied by the corresponding weight to yield a number of quality-adjusted life-years.

Many methods have been used to measure these weights [33–36] with varying results. Hamel et al. based their cost-utility analysis on the group of patients in the Study to Understand Prognoses and Preferences for Outcomes and Risks of Treatment (SUPPORT) with pneumonia or acute respiratory distress syndrome (ARDS) who received mechanical ventilation. The cost per QALY was US$ 29 000 for patients with a greater than 70% probability of surviving two months but US$ 110 000 for patients with a less than 50% probability of surviving two months [37]. These costs are much greater than Australian estimates of between A$297 for patients with asthma to A$2323 for patients with pulmonary oedema treated in intensive care, though the methods used were substantially different [38].

Cost-Benefit Analysis

Cost-benefit analysis recognises the multidimensional nature of health outcomes but unlike cost-utility analysis, the consequences are valued in monetary units providing a means to compare costs and consequences directly. Methods include the human-capital approach and the willingness-to-pay approach [39] with the willingness-to-pay approach (i.e., the maximum amount of money that an individual is willing to pay for a specific outcome or course of action) being the most common.

The Cost of Benefit

Determining the cost of benefit for intensive care is difficult, though this is not unique to intensive care. The American Thoracic Society (2002) [40] identified several issues that hamper cost-effectiveness analyses including:

- Lack of information on the effectiveness of ICU interventions
- ICU patients are complex, with multiple concurrent problems and interventions
- Most ICU therapies are only supportive, and therefore may not individually result in improved outcome
- Accurate costs commonly are not available and they are difficult to obtain
- No standardised approach for measuring or valuing costs across countries
- Preferred outcomes for cost-effectiveness analyses such as long-term quality-adjusted survival are rarely available
- Valuing the importance of appropriate end-of-life care, an important aspect of ICU care, is difficult
- The burden of critical illness on family members is not easily captured in a cost-effectiveness analysis

In cost-effectiveness studies of intensive care the cost per year of life gained varies considerably and studies are limited by duration and loss to follow up [41, 42]. These studies assumed all patients would have died if not admitted to the ICU. This assumption is vulnerable. Even when intensive care was considered futile because of chronic disease and acute illness severity, 10% of patients survived to leave hospital without intensive care [43] and survival was even greater in less severely ill patients refused intensive care admission. As an alternative to assuming that all patients would have died without intensive care, two studies [37, 44] have compared outcomes in patients who had intensive care withdrawn or withheld, with patients who continued to be treated. Survival among patients who had care limited was between 0 and 10%. However, this still represents an invalid comparison group, as patients who have treatment limited will be systematically different to the group in which treatment is continued, with higher severity of illness and more co-morbidities.

Although intensive care is said to be expensive when compared to other health services, Sznajder et al. [42] demonstrated a moderate cost benefit for intensive care units.

Measuring Costs

Costs can be calculated by several different ways and comparison of costs is complex [45]. No system adequately costs intensive care services [46]. Part of the difficulty is that intensive care is usually only part of an episode of care and may not be costed or funded separately. Intensive care unit costs may be buried in the overall cost of a hospital admission. However, all costs directly incurred as a result of providing healthcare should be included in an economic evaluation [30].

Direct Costs

These should include the 'up-front' costs associated with the implementation of the intervention (i.e., nurse and physician wages, etc.) as well as 'downstream' costs of resources consumed in the future that are still attributable to the intervention (depending on the viewpoint). When costs are directly calculated, the cost figures do not represent the same cost components [24]. In studies where the intensive care unit management or outcome is the priority or where the costs of different intensive care units are compared, only direct costs, that is, those costs directly attributed to the functioning of the ICU rather than overhead costs, are relevant [2, 24, 46, 47].

Indirect Costs

In addition to direct costs, costs to the patient (time off from work, child care, travel, etc.), costs borne by employers, other employees, society, and non-health aspects of the intervention on society should be considered from a societal perspective [48].

Costing Methods

Methods of costing patient care in the ICU include averaging costs from dividing total annual expenditure by patient throughput [11, 49], the use of severity of illness and workload scoring systems [21, 50, 51] and the use of billing systems [52]. The diversity of costing methods has resulted in poor external validity and inability to compare findings [24]. The measures of cost and outcome need to be accurate and reproducible if these costing studies are to be of any value [29]. Studies often have identified the costs of intensive care in isolation, without considering their application and validity in the strategic planning and management of services [53].

Total Annual Expenditure By Patient Throughput

The total cost of intensive care has been estimated from the cost of ICU care per day and the national number of ICU days [11]. Data is often abstracted from administrative databases, and it seems reasonable to presume that these data are approximately accurate [11, 23]. The validity of this estimate is difficult to judge, but it is unlikely to overestimate costs and subsequent work using a cost accounting method suggests it underestimates costs by 20 to 30% [54].

However, using the average bed/day price and multiplying this with length of stay per patient to calculate the intensive care costs per patient does not reflect patient-specific resource use [24]. It assumes that the resource use is constant during the entire stay in the unit, which is inappropriate. The first hours after admission to an intensive care unit may be very resource-intensive but after these initial activities resource use is not uniform. Some patients quickly become stabilised requiring fewer resources while other patients require more and more resources. The assumption of a constant cost per day makes it impossible to study the relationship between costs, therapeutic activity, and outcome, as costs only depend on length of stay and have no empirical or theoretical relation to other factors that influence resource use [24].

Charges

Charges are often used as surrogates for 'costs'. The relationship between charges and costs is weak and not an appropriate method to study ICU costs [9, 24, 46]. Charges almost always reflect something different to the actual resources consumed [52]. Charges (and cost-to-charge ratios) are specific to a particular institution and may even vary within an institution depending on the payer and the insurance coverage and thus are likely to lack generalisability [30]. Different patient groups cannot be compared using costs based on estimated hospital charges because they frequently rely on average costs or charges [25].

Total charges, weighted length of stay and a computerised Therapeutic Intervention Scoring System (TISS), adapted from the Therapeutic Intervention Scoring System [55] correlated closely with costs [56]. This method was validated in another institution and showed high internal validity [57]. Weighted length of stay was considered by the authors as a valuable measure of costs because of its high performance, simplicity and wide availability. However, the costs included in different hospital billing systems may vary and may not take into account all the costs associated with a patient's care. For example, they do not include costs for medical staff. Acknowledging that charges do not reflect actual costs, a cost-to-charge index may be used to adjust the charges but it is difficult to ascertain what the final cost figure actually represents [24].

Routine calculation of the cost of an individual ICU patient is feasible using a computerised patient data management system that stores all the activities of care delivered to an individual patient [53]. The activity-based costing methodology determines the patient-related or direct costs of care for individual patients. The total costs of care for an individual patient are the sum of the patient related costs of care and a proportion of the non-patient-related costs associated with running the ICU. It ignores hospital overheads. It was not possible to ascertain how the cost of each activity was determined from this study report. The non-patient-related costs such as rates, utilities and energy were calculated by apportioning the total hospital bill by the percentage of floor area that the ICU occupies. Nevertheless, it is a useful costing model. Such sophisticated information systems are not available in many ICUs.

Lack of Standardisation

Although economic evaluations are increasingly common there are no standardised methods to measure or value costs. A diversity of costing methods has resulted in poor external validity and an inability to compare findings between such evaluations [24]. Typical outcomes in ICU studies (for example short-term mortality) are not ideal for cost effective analysis studies while preferred outcomes for cost effective analysis studies (for example, long-term quality-adjusted survival) are limited by the lack of long-term outcome data for patients treated with intensive care [40]. A comprehensive review of economic evaluations in intensive care identified only 6 out of 29 studies which measured and valued costs appropriately [58]. A review of 20 studies that estimated costs in adult intensive care concluded that all of the many methods used were flawed [24].

A detailed Australian study of 100 consecutive patients admitted to a tertiary hospital ICU in 1983 estimated mean ICU cost per admission to be $1357 but the variation is reflected by a standard deviation of $2676 [45]. These cost estimates excluded equipment capital costs and maintenance, and the hospital building and overhead costs. Labour costs accounted for 54% of the total. An activity based costing method [59] estimated overhead costs to be almost half the total average daily cost for intensive care but there were large variations in individual patient related costs. This estimate of non-patient related cost is at the upper end of those reported. Differences in costing methods preclude the generalisability of studies [58].

A standardised method that could be considered as the 'gold standard' for costing intensive care is essential to ensure valid dissemination and implementation of cost-effective measures [27]. While Glydmark [24] and Heyland et al. [58] concluded a standardised model is needed for costing intensive care, such a model has yet to be agreed or widely used. The *Recommendations for reporting cost-effectiveness analyses* state that a complete description of estimates of resource use and effectiveness should be provided with the methods used for obtaining estimates of costs and effectiveness and the results of sensitivity analyses [60]. The *Recommendations* do not advocate a specific model or models for deriving cost estimates.

Information on what constitutes the costs and cost-effectiveness is limited [27] with only a small number of economic evaluations to identify how intensive care resources could be used more effectively [28, 40]. Although intensive care is widely accepted as effective, this cannot be accurately quantified because of the absence of clinical trials in which admission to the ICU is randomised. In the absence of objective evidence, most studies make overly pessimistic assumptions about outcome without intensive care.

Differing unit prices for doctors' fees, nurses' wages, pharmaceuticals, laboratory tests, etc., will result in a different mix of resources consumed to perform the same task. Differing patient volumes will result in different average and/or marginal costs across centres. Converting costs using exchange rates between countries represents a formidable challenge because exchange rates do not, in most cases, reflect the relative difference in costs of resources consumed; rather, they reflect government monetary policy [30].

Standardisation of methods will improve the comparability of the results of economic evaluations of various healthcare interventions, but it will not eliminate the problems associated with generalising results to other settings due to differences in healthcare systems [58].

Sensitivity Analysis

Uncertainty in many economic analyses arises from lack of precision of clinical or cost estimates, from methodological weaknesses in the data used, or from lack of empirical data [30]. To deal with uncertainty, a sensitivity analysis may be performed. Estimates of effectiveness and cost (even from weak data or data derived from the consensus of experts) should be incorporated into a sensitivity analysis to determine over what range of assumptions the results remain stable [30]. The estimates should be varied through a range of plausible values to determine what effect this has on the conclusions of the economic analysis [30]. If, despite varying key estimates (either of effectiveness or costs), the conclusions remain the same, they can be considered robust but if the recommendations of the economic evaluation change when key variables are altered, it may be difficult to accept the inferences from the analysis [30].

Sensitivity analysis has not been widely used to estimate the range of cost-effectiveness associated with different assumptions about outcome in intensive care [58]. Sensitivity analyses can be used to deal with problems of generalisability, since underlying assumptions can be varied to see what impact they have on the overall results [58].

Valuation of Costs and Outcomes

The valuation of costs and consequences should be adjusted for differences in their timing. Because as individuals, and as a society, we typically prefer to have dollars or benefits now as opposed to later, future costs and benefits are adjusted or reduced (i.e., discounted) to reflect the fact that, for example, dollars saved or spent in the future are not valued as highly as dollars spent or saved today. Although there is general agreement that costs and consequences that occur in the future should be discounted to present values, there is no agreement on the discount rate [61]. The rate is dependent on the local healthcare system and the viewpoint of the analysis [61].

Macro- and Micro-Economics

Costs can be evaluated at the macro or micro economic level. As health care costs continue to rise, most developed countries have developed strategies for controlling their health care budgets. Considering the high-cost, low-throughput of the ICU, it is natural to examine and justify utilisation of critical care resources [44, 62]. Despite estimates, neither the true costs of intensive care or its benefits in terms of cost are known [2, 23] and few of the specific interventions that form a part of intensive care have been subject to cost-effectiveness analysis [63].

International Cost Comparisons for Intensive Care Services

Although the cost of ICU care per day is similar in most countries, the number of ICU beds differs substantially. Comparing the cost of intensive care is difficult because the definition and provision of services varies [4, 25]. The definition of intensive care varies between countries and may include or exclude coronary care beds, high-dependency beds, neonatal beds, and other specific bed types when ICU bed numbers are counted. ICU beds in Australia are commonly reported per head of population and as a percentage of total hospital beds [64]. An international comparison of the ratio of ICU to hospital beds and the number of ICU beds per capita are shown in Table 1.

Intensive care resource use also varies between different patient groups including age, sex, and race, independent of severity of primary disease [65–68]. For example, fewer resources are reportedly used on the elderly

[69–77] or women when compared to men [78]. The cost for patients with higher levels of severity of illness and needing mechanical ventilation are greater than those who do not need mechanical ventilation [79–81]. Therefore ICUs with a higher proportion of ventilated patients will incur more costs.

International Comparison of Critical Care Services

The United States

Healthcare costs in the United States have increased rapidly in the past few decades [82], reaching US$1.37 trillion in 2001 [83] despite a shift in United States health care delivery from in-patient- to out-patient-based care [23] that was predicted to decrease hospital costs [84]. It was estimated that more than 20% of hospital budgets were used on the care of intensive care patients, representing approximately 1% of the gross national product [16, 85]. Patients receiving intensive care accounted for nearly 30% of acute care hospital costs, yet occupied only 10% of inpatient beds [16, 86]. However, these estimates are based on outdated reports [11, 16, 87].

A recent study found that, despite its increasing use and cost, critical care is using proportionally less of United States national health expenses and the gross domestic product than previously estimated [23]. Critical care was defined as intensive care unit, coronary care unit, burn intensive care unit, surgical intensive care unit, and other special care units. Between 1985 and 2000, using the United States federal sector's Hospital Cost Report Information System (HCRIS) data analyses and Russell equation cost calculations [11, 16], the number of acute care hospital beds decreased but the absolute and proportional number of critical care beds increased [16]. The number of United States hospitals with critical care beds decreased by 13.7%, but the number of critical care beds increased by 26.2% and critical care bed costs per day increased by 126% (US$1,185 to US$2,674). This contrasts to the decrease in total hospital beds of 26.4%.

Although overall United States health expenditures rose by more than 200%, critical care costs increased by 190% (US$19.1 billion to US$55.5 billion), the proportion of national health expenditures for critical care decreasing by 5.4%. In 2000, critical care costs represented 13.3% of hospital costs, 4.2% of national health expenditures, and 0.56% of the gross domestic product [23]. The relative increase in the costs of ward admission and escalating costs for pharmaceuticals (both inpatient and outpatient) may explain why proportionally ICU care costs have decreased over time [26]. The data were not corrected for changes in the consumer price index (CPI) or inflation.

The United States is not typical of other healthcare systems because over-use and oversupply of technology combined in some cases with poorer out-comes and difficulties containing costs have resulted in a very different healthcare delivery system [64].

The United Kingdom

United Kingdom ICUs have a lower intensive care to acute hospital bed ratio than most Western European countries [4]. The cost of adult ICUs in the United Kingdom has been estimated as UK£700 million, which represents only 0.1% of GDP [4]. In the United Kingdom costs are rising at about 5 to 10% per year, which is substantially above the rate of general medical infla-tion, although this appreciation is from a low base by international compari-son [4]. The average individual cost per patient day in the United Kingdom was estimated to be UK£1152 including an allowance for overheads [53].

Australia and New Zealand

In 2001 there were 172 ICUs in Australia with 1272 beds which admitted 137 598 patients [88]. It is likely that Australian and New Zealand costs for intensive care lie between the United States and the United Kingdom figures, though probably closer to United Kingdom levels. However, a total cost is not available for either country.

Comparing outcome and performance between different countries and different intensive care units is difficult because of enormous variations in case mix, severity of illness, co-morbidities, social expectations, medical cul-ture and recording methods [89, 90]. In the intensive care unit context, illness severity is likely to be the major determinant of outcome and but not neces-sarily of cost. The highest cost patients tend to be those with a high illness severity, so they are not expected to survive, and patients with a low illness severity on admission who develop complications from which they die. Severity standardisation of patients with critical illness has proved difficult [17]. There are a number of severity scoring systems; all have limitations and none are universally accepted.

Estimation of Patient-Specific Costs

Only a few studies measure patient-specific costs, with the majority focusing on costs averaged across all patients [29]. Little is known about the factors that influence individual patient cost variation [24]. Patient-specific costs define resources that can be directly attributed to an individual patient. These would include the costs of drugs and disposables used by that patient, laboratory tests, blood and blood products as well as medical and nursing time spent directly on patient care. These resources account for the majority of costs, with the remainder usually considered as 'overheads'. It is necessary to measure patient-specific costs to determine what influences them [29].

The cost block method, with precise definitions for cost collection [25], demonstrated considerable variability in several areas of ICU expenditure between different ICUs [27, 29]. Adjusting total expenditure, by the size of the ICU, patient throughput, hospital type and the presence of a high-dependency unit, some of the variation in costs was explained and in greater detail than previously reported [27, 29]. Multivariate analysis showed that 93% of the variation in expenditure on disposable equipment could be explained by the number of ICU beds, the number of admissions and the presence of a high-dependency unit, 92% of the variation in nursing staff expenditure was explained by the number of ICU beds and the presence of an high-dependency unit, 76% of the variation in expenditure on consultant staff was explained by hospital type and the number of patient days whilst 64% of the variation in drug and fluid expenditure was explained by the number of patient days [27].

Studies have identified several variables as predictors of daily cost: medical versus surgical patients [1, 91]; diagnosis [54, 92]; the Acute Physiology and Chronic Health Evaluation (APACHE) II severity score [53, 80]; elective or emergency admission [54, 92]; clinical severity [45]; workload units [53, 92]; mechanical ventilation [80]; length of ICU stay [53] and survival [1, 54, 80, 91, 92].

The reported costs per patient vary widely [24, 93]. Reasons for this may include [24]:

– Technological changes have affected costs in both a negative and a positive way.
– Patients vary between studies with regard to healthcare needs, severity of illness, age, diagnosis, and other characteristics. Some units treat only medical patients, while other units treat surgical patients or both types of patients. Patient case mix and variation in severity of illness should be adjusted in order to compare results across studies.
– Unit characteristics such as unit size, staffing, treatment policies, and research and training activities may differ widely and thus influence costs
– Possibilities for treatment and care in the various units may be very different, and may thereby contribute to diversities in both the selection of patients treated and the therapeutic activity of the unit. Intensive care units that use state of the art equipment to provide more services may increase the cost of treatment (and improve outcome).
– The method for costing services varies widely leading to methodological bias which may not reflect actual differences.

What the literature often fails to acknowledge is that intensive care units tend to care for the sickest patients, irrespective of admitting diagnosis. These patients are a heterogeneous group and display a wide variability in terms of severity of illness and patient acuity. Intuitively, cost-effectiveness should vary according to case-mix and acuity but most economic studies in critical care neglect this, grouping patients together [2].

The limited information on the cost-effectiveness of intensive care is, therefore, based on few studies with small cohorts of patients, most often in selected patient populations, with insufficient duration of patient follow-up, overly optimistic assumptions about the effectiveness of ICU, and an absence of agreed costing methods. The wide range of reported values for cost-effectiveness and cost-utility are reflective of the use of different methods. There is a need for cost-effectiveness analysis for adult intensive care over a range of effectiveness assumptions using long-term follow-up and with modern costings.

Reducing Costs

There has been increasing emphasis on developing ways to slow the rate of growth of increasing healthcare costs including avoiding the need for intensive care, decreasing length of stay, analysis of costs in various subgroups of patients, minimising utilisation of unnecessary treatments, and limiting life-sustaining therapy for those who may not benefit from it [9]. Although using age as a criterion for making decisions about medical care is controversial, surveys of physicians and the public have indicated an acceptance of limiting life-sustaining therapy based on age [94–97].

Length of Stay

ICU length of stay is a simple measure to assess resource utilisation. ICU cost per day can be assumed to be consistent across most diagnoses [54] and has been used as a surrogate measure of ICU resource utilisation [89, 98–100]. Reducing ICU length of stay has been thought to improve efficiency [101, 102] and has been achieved through the use of clinical pathways, protocols and care maps. Length of stay however, is affected by factors that are unique to individual patients which cannot be changed [103]. Although there has been a global trend to reduce hospital length of stay, no change in ICU length of stay was observed in the United States from 1988 to 1996 [104]. Elderly patients who died in ICU had lower hospital charges than did younger non-survivors but there was little difference in lengths of stay [70]. Most of the costs are due to care of the small number of patients who receive intensive care for longer than 5-7 days [5].

High-Cost Patients

Large resources in the ICU are devoted to patients with a poor prognosis, many of whom ultimately die [29, 105, 106]. Predicting high-cost patients with poor survival might reduce costs. A small percentage of hospitalised patients consume a large proportion of the total available hospital resources [107–109]. There have been few studies [110–112] to identify specific patient groups whose quality of life remains poor [112–114] or the longer term prognosis of those patients who are the major consumers of intensive care resources [115]. No prognostic system has been developed that accurately identifies an individuals' survival or future quality of life.

In an Australian study into costs, severity of illness and outcomes in one hundred ICU patients, there was no evidence to suggest any association between costs and subsequent quality of life of survivors [45]. There was a strong association between survival and total admission costs confirming 'high risk is high cost'. Although this study was conducted several years ago and the follow-up time was only for one month after ICU discharge, it is one of the few studies that has measured direct ICU costs using an appropriate and accurate costing method that is still relevant.

To control the excess in healthcare costs over the long-term, it is necessary to address the decisions physicians make about treatments [116]. Understanding and altering factors that influence clinical decision-making has a high likelihood of impacting on the volume and intensity of services. Treatment decisions are based largely, but not exclusively, on: a) the clinical consequences of treatment (i.e., the clinical benefits compared with the risks or adverse effects); b) the economic consequences of treatment (i.e., the benefits relative to the costs); or c) some combination of both the clinical and economic consequences [58].

Patient preferences for treatments and outcomes are of great importance to ICU decision-making, especially when evaluating the trade-off between quality and quantity of life. To live longer but neurologically impaired may not be as desirable as living for a shorter period in full health, or not living at all. Yet there are no economic evaluations that include data on patient preferences [58].

Conclusions

Costing studies are needed for appropriate allocation of scarce health care resources to areas where the greatest benefit can be achieved in terms of both survival and quality of life [117–119]. However, the consistency and quality of cost studies in intensive care are problematic, hampering quality research and economic planning [120, 121]. The methods have often been flawed and fail to provide correct answers [24]. Moreover, the costing methods applied in many studies are wrongly specified in relation to the purpose and viewpoint of these studies [24]. Using standardised models for determining intensive care unit costs will improve intensive care unit costing studies [24, 25, 42, 56]. Despite their complexity, a standardised costing model will facilitate better, faster, and more reliable costings, improving quality, facilitating best practice, proving comparability of studies, and their ultimate utility [24, 48, 53, 120, 122].

Improving efficiency should significantly reduce costs [123]. Intensivists are becoming more cost-conscious and increasingly demand evidence of cost-effectiveness before new interventions and technologies are adopted [26]. However, the lack of clinically applicable cost-accounting models which reflect the true costs of care currently limit the possibility of demonstrating cost-effectiveness in intensive care [12].

The perception of intensive care as a costly speciality is based on a purely accounting approach [42]. The allocation of resources should be related to outcomes in performance including long term survival, quality of life after intensive care unit care and patient preferences [48].

Table 1. International comparison of the ratio of ICU to hospital beds and the number of ICU beds per capita

Country	Ratio ICU: hospital beds	ICU beds/million
England and Wales	1 to 2% [4]	41/million [4]
US	13.4%* [23]	310*/million [23]
Australia	3 to 4% [124]	75/million [124]
Germany	2.7% [125]	280/million[125]
France	3.2% [125]	380/million [125]

*total critical care beds including intensive care beds, coronary care beds, burns

References

1. Norris C, Jacobs P, Rapoport J et al (1995) ICU and non-ICU cost per day. Can J Anaest 42(3):192–196
2. Chalfin DB, Cohen IL, Lambrinos J (1995) The economics and cost-effectiveness of critical care medicine. Intensive Care Med 21(11):952–961
3. Chelluri L, Im KA, Belle SH et al (2004) Long-term mortality and quality of life after prolonged mechanical ventilation. Crit Care Med 32(1):61–69
4. Audit Commission, for Local Authorities, & NHS in, England, Wales (1999) Critical to Success. The place of efficient and effective critical care services within the acute hospital. London
5. Parviainen I, Herranen A, Holm A et al (2004) Results and costs of intensive care in a tertiary university hospital from 1996-2000. Acta Anaesthesiol Scand 48(1):55–60
6. Spillman BC, Lubitz J (2000) The effect of longevity on spending for acute and long-

term care. N Engl J Med 342(19):1409–1415

7. Lubitz J, Greenberg LG, Gorina Y et al (2001) Three decades of health care use by the elderly, 1965-1998. Health Aff 20(2):19–32

8. Rubenfeld GD, Angus DC, Pinsky MR et al (1999) Outcomes research in critical care: results of the American Thoracic Society Critical Care Assembly Workshop on Outcomes Research. The Members of the Outcomes Research Workshop. Am J Respir Crit Care Med 160(1):358–367

9. Chelluri L, Grenvik A, Silverman M (1995) Intensive care for critically ill elderly: mortality, costs, and quality of life. Review of the literature. Arch Intern Med 155(10):1013–1022

10. Kvåle R, Flaatten H (2002) Changes in intensive care from 1987 to 1997 - has outcome improved? A single centre study. Intensive Care Med 28(8):1110–1116

11. Jacobs P, Noseworthy TW (1990) National estimates of intensive care utilization and costs: Canada and the United States. Crit Care Med 18(11):1282–1286

12. Buist M (1994) Intensive care unit resource utilisation. Anaesth Intensive Care 22(1):46–60

13. Cerra FB (1993) Healthcare reform: the role of coordinated critical care. Crit Care Med 21(3):457–464

14. Cullen DJ (1977) Results and costs of intensive care. Anesthesiology 47(2):203–216

15. Fakhry SM, Kercher KW, Rutledge R (1996) Survival, quality of life, and charges in critically III surgical patients requiring prolonged ICU stays. J Trauma 41(6):999–1007

16. Halpern NA, Bettes L, Greenstein R (1994) Federal and nationwide intensive care units and healthcare costs: 1986-1992. Crit Care Med 22(12):2001–2007

17. Henderson A (1997) Adult intensive care in an environment of resource restriction: how should the unit director respond? Aust Health Rev 20(2):68–82

18. Singer M, Myers S, Hall G et al (1994) The cost of intensive care: a comparison on one unit between 1988 and 1991. Intensive Care Med 20(8):542–549

19. Becker GJ, Strauch GO, Saranchak HJ (1984) Outcome and cost of prolonged stay in the surgical intensive care unit. Arch Surg 119(11):1338–1342

20. Cullen DJ, Keene R, Waternaux C et al (1984) Results, charges, and benefits of intensive care for critically ill patients: update 1983. Crit Care Med 12(2):102–106

21. Loes O, Smith-Erichsen N, Lind B (1987) Intensive care: cost and benefit. Acta Anaesthesiol Scand 84(Suppl):3–19

22. Spicher JE, White DP (1987) Outcome and function following prolonged mechanical ventilation. Arch Intern Med 147(3):421–425

23. Halpern NA, Pastores SM, Greenstein RJ (2004) Critical Care Medicine in the United States 1985-2000: An analysis of bed numbers, use, and costs. Crit Care Med 32(6):1254–1259

24. Gyldmark M (1995) A review of cost studies of intensive care units: problems with the cost concept. Crit Care Med 23(5):964–972

25. Edbrooke D, Hibbert C, Ridley S et al (1999) The development of a method for comparative costing of individual intensive care units. The Intensive Care Working Group on Costing. Anaesthesia 54(2):110–120

26. Shorr AF, Linde-Zwirble WT, Angus DC (2004) No longer the 'expensive scare unit'? Crit Care Med 32(6):1408–1409

27. Edbrooke DL, Ridley SA, Hibbert CL, Corcoran M (2001) Variations in expenditure between adult general intensive care units in the UK. Anaesthesia 56(3):208–216

28. Chalfin DB (1998) Evidence-based medicine and cost-effectiveness analysis. Critical Care Clinics 14(3):525–537

29. Jacobs P, Edbrooke D, Hibbert C et al (2001) Descriptive patient data as an explanation for the variation in average daily costs in intensive care. Anaesthesia 56(7):643–647

30. Heyland DK, Gafni A, Kernerman P et al (1999) How to use the results of an economic evaluation. Crit Care Med 27(6):1195–1202

31. Gafni A (1996) Economic evaluation of health care interventions: an economist's perspective. ACP J Club 124(2):A12–A4

32. Elliott D (1997) Costing intensive care services: a review of study methods, results and limitations. Australian Critical Care 10(2):55–63

33. Drummond MF (1987) Economic evaluation and the rational diffusion and use of health technology. Health Policy 7(3):309–324

34. O'Brien BJ, Heyland D, Richardson WS et al (1997) Users' guides to the medical literature. XIII. How to use an article on economic analysis of clinical practice. B. What are the results and will they help me in caring for my patients? Evidence-Based Medicine Working Group. JAMA 277(22):1802–1806

35. Gafni A (1994) The standard gamble method: what is being measured and how it is interpreted. Health Serv Res 29(2):207–224

36. Mehrez A, Gafni A (1992) Preference based outcome measures for economic evaluation of drug interventions: quality adjusted life years (QALYs) versus healthy years equivalents (HYEs). Pharmacoeconomics 1(5):338–345

37. Hamel MB, Phillips RS, Davis RB et al (2000) Outcomes and cost-effectiveness of ventilator support and aggressive care for patients with acute respiratory failure due to pneumonia or acute respiratory distress syndrome. Am J Med 109(8):614–620

38. Kerridge RK, Glasziou PP, Hillman KM (1995) The use of 'quality-adjusted life years' (QALYs) to evaluate treatment in intensive care. Anaesth Intensive Care 23(3):322–331

39. Gafni A (1997) Willingness to pay in the context of an economic evaluation of healthcare programs: theory and practice. Am J Manag Care 3(Suppl):S21-S32

40. Anonymous (2002) Understanding costs and cost-effectiveness in critical care: report from the second American Thoracic Society workshop on outcomes research. Am J Respir Crit Care Med 165(4):540–550

41. Vang J, Karlsson P, Hakansson S (1985) Intensive care for the aged in a Swedish community hospital. A cost-effectiveness analysis. In: International Journal of Technology Assessment in Health Care, pp 893–900

42. Sznajder M, Aegerter P, Launois R et al (2001) A cost-effectiveness analysis of stays in intensive care units. Intensive Care Med 27(1):146–153

43. Joynt GM, Gomersall CD, Tan P et al (2001) Prospective evaluation of patients refused admission to an intensive care unit: triage, futility and outcome. Intensive Care Med 27(9):1459–1465

44. Heyland DK, Konopad E, Noseworthy TW et al (1998) Is it 'worthwhile' to continue treating patients with a prolonged stay (>14 days) in the ICU? An economic evaluation. Chest 114(1):192–198

45. Slatyer MA, James OF, Moore PG, Leeder SR (1986) Costs, severity of illness and outcome in intensive care. Anaesth Intensive Care 14(4):381–389

46. Jegers M (1997) Cost accounting in ICUs: beneficial for management and research. Intensive Care Med 23(6):618–619

47. Shiell AM, Griffiths RD, Short AI, Spiby J (1990) An evaluation of the costs and outcome of adult intensive care in two units in the UK. Clin Intensive Care 1(6):256–262

48. Weinstein MC, Siegel JE, Gold MR et al (1996) Recommendations of the Panel on Cost-effectiveness in Health and Medicine. JAMA 276(15):1253–1258

49. Byrick R, Mindorff C, McKee L et al (1980) Cost-effectiveness of intensive care for respiratory failure patients. Crit Care Med 8(6):332–337

50. Atkinson S, Bihari D, Smithies M et al (1994) Identification of futility in intensive care. Lancet 344(8931):1203–1206

51. Zimmerman JE, Shortell SM, Knaus WA et al (1993) Value and cost of teaching hospitals: a prospective, multicenter, inception cohort study. Crit Care Med 21(10):1432–1442

52. Finkler S (1982) The distinction between cost and charges. Ann Intern Med 96(1):102–109

53. Edbrooke DL, Stevens VG, Hibbert CL et al (1997) A new method of accurately identifying costs of individual patients in intensive care: the initial results. Intensive Care Med 23(6):645–650

54. Noseworthy TW, Konopad E, Shustack A et al (1996) Cost accounting of adult intensive care: methods and human and capital inputs. Crit Care Med 24(7):1168–1172

55. Cullen DJ, Civetta JM, Briggs BA, Ferrara LC (1974) Therapeutic intervention scoring system: a method for quantitative comparison of patient care. Crit Care Med 2(2):57–60

56. Clermont G, Angus D, Linde-Zwirble W et al (1996) Alternative measures of ICU resource use: do they compare? Crit Care Med 24(S1):A52

57. Herr D, Clermont G, Angus D (1998) Generating TISS-28 scores directly from hospital billing data. Validation on new hospital data. Crit Care Med 26:A66

58. Heyland DK, Kernerman P, Gafni A, Cook DJ (1996) Economic evaluations in the critical care literature: do they help us improve the efficiency of our unit? Crit Care Med 24(9):1591–1598

59. Edbrooke DL, Stevens VG, Hibbert CL et al (1997) A new method of accurately identifying costs of individual patients in intensive care: the initial results. Intensive Care Med 23:645–650

60. Siegel JE, Weinstein MC, Russell LB, Gold MR (1996) Recommendations for reporting cost-effectiveness analyses. Panel on Cost-Effectiveness in Health and Medicine. JAMA 276(16):1339–1341

61. Krahn M, Gafni A (1993) Discounting in the economic evaluation of health care interventions. Medical Care 31(5):403–418

62. Bion JF, Bennett D (1999) Epidemiology of Intensive Care Med: supply versus demand. British Medical Bulletin 55(1):2–11

63. Shorr AF (2002) An update on cost-effectiveness analysis in critical care. Curr Opin Crit Care 8(4):337–343

64. Anonymous (1997) Acute Health Division DoHS. Review of intensive care in Victoria (Phase 1 report). Melbourne Department of Human Services

65. Epstein AM, Ayanian JZ, Keogh JH et al (2000) Racial disparities in access to renal transplantation—clinically appropriate or due to underuse or overuse? N Engl J Med 343(21):1537–1544

66. Rathore SS, Berger AK, Weinfurt KP et al (2000) Race, sex, poverty, and the medical treatment of acute myocardial infarction in the elderly. Circulation 102(6):642–648

67. Gan SC, Beaver SK, Houck PM et al (2000) Treatment of acute myocardial infarction and 30-day mortality among women and men. N Engl J Med 343(1):8–15

68. Buckle JM, Horn SD, Oates VM, Abbey H (1992) Severity of illness and resource use differences among white and black hospitalized elderly. Archives of Internal Medicine 152(8):1596–1603

69. Chalfin DB, Carlon GC (1990) Age and utilization of intensive care unit resources of critically ill cancer patients. Crit Care Med 18(7):694–698

70. Campion EW, Mulley AG, Goldstein RL et al (1981) Medical intensive care for the elderly. A study of current use, costs, and outcomes. JAMA 246(18):2052–2056
71. Hamel MB, Phillips RS, Teno JM et al (1996) Seriously ill hospitalized adults: do we spend less on older patients? Support Investigators. Study to Understand Prognoses and Preference for Outcomes and Risks of Treatments. J Am Geriatr Soc 44(9):1043–1048
72. Hamel MB, Teno JM, Goldman L et al (1999) Patient age and decisions to withhold life-sustaining treatments from seriously ill, hospitalized adults. SUPPORT Investigators. Study to Understand Prognoses and Preferences for Outcomes and Risks of Treatment. Annals of Internal Medicine 130(2):116–125
73. Hamel MB, Davis RB, Teno JM et al (1999) Older age, aggressiveness of care, and survival for seriously ill, hospitalized adults. SUPPORT Investigators. Study to Understand Prognoses and Preferences for Outcomes and Risks of Treatments. Annals of Internal Medicine 131(10):721–728
74. Perls TT, Wood ER (1996) Acute care costs of the oldest old: they cost less, their care intensity is less, and they go to nonteaching hospitals. Archives of Internal Medicine 156(7):754–760
75. Boyd K, Teres D, Rapoport J, Lemeshow S (1996) The relationship between age and the use of DNR orders in critical care patients. Evidence for age discrimination. Arch Intern Med 156(16):1821–1826
76. Ely EW, Evans GW, Haponik EF (1999) Mechanical ventilation in a cohort of elderly patients admitted to an intensive care unit. Ann Intern Med 131(2):96–104
77. Angus DC, Linde-Zwirble WT, Lidicker J et al (2001) Epidemiology of severe sepsis in the United States: analysis of incidence, outcome, and associated costs of care. Crit Care Med 29(7):1303–1310
78. Valentin A, Jordan B, Lang T et al (2003) Gender-related differences in intensive care: a multiple-center cohort study of therapeutic interventions and outcome in critically ill patients. Crit Care Med 31(7):1901–1907
79. Wagner DP (1989) Economics of prolonged mechanical ventilation. Am Rev Respir Dis 140(2 Pt 2):S14–S8
80. Ridley S, Biggam M, Stone P (1991) Cost of intensive therapy. A description of methodology and initial results. Anaesthesia 46(7):523–530
81. Rapoport J, Teres D, Lemeshow S et al (1990) Explaining variability of cost using a severity-of-illness measure for ICU patients. Med Care 28(4):338–348
82. Cowan CA, Lazenby HC, Martin AB et al (2001) National health expenditures, 1999. Health Care Financ Rev 22(4):77–110
83. Anonymous (2004) United States Census Bureau. Statistical Abstract of the United States: 2003. Chapter 3 Health and Nutrition. In: http://www.census.gov/prod/www/statistical-abstract-04.html
84. Aiken LH, Clarke SP, Sloane DM (2001) Hospital restructuring: does it adversely affect care and outcomes? J Health Hum Serv Adm 23(4):416–442
85. Esserman L, Belkora J, Lenert L (1995) Potentially ineffective care. A new outcome to assess the limits of critical care. JAMA 274(19):1544–1551
86. Anonymous (1994) Joint position statement: essential provisions for critical care in health system reform. Society of Crit Care Med. American Association of Critical Care Nurses. Crit Care Med 22(12):2017–2019
87. Groeger JS, Guntupalli KK, Strosberg M et al (1993) Descriptive analysis of critical care units in the United States: patient characteristics and intensive care unit utilization. Crit Care Med 21(2):279–291
88. Clarke T, Hart LG (2002) Review of ICU Resorces & Activity 00/01. In: Australian &

New Zealand Intensive Care Society

89. Knaus WA, Wagner DP, Zimmerman JE, Draper EA (1993) Variations in mortality and length of stay in intensive care units. Annals of Internal Medicine 118(10):753–761

90. Zimmerman JE, Knaus WA, Judson JA et al (1988) Patient selection for intensive care: a comparison of New Zealand and United States hospitals. Crit Care Med 16(4):318–326

91. Parno JR, Teres D, Lemeshow S et al (1982) Hospital charges and long-term survival of ICU versus non-ICU patients. Crit Care Med 10(9):569–574

92. Girotti MJ, Brown SJ (1986) Reducing the costs of ICU admission in Canada without diagnosis–related or case-mix groupings. Canadian Anaesthetists' Society Journal 33(6):765–772

93. Surgenor S, Mroz W, Henry S et al (1998) Cost of hospital care for selected diagnosis related groups with and without intensive care unit admission. Crit Care Med 26:42A

94. Williams A, Evans JG (1997) The rationing debate. Rationing health care by age. BMJ 314(7083):820–825

95. Williams M (1997) Rationing health care. Can a 'fair innings' ever be fair? BMJ 314(7079):15

96. Bowling A (1996) Health care rationing: the public's debate. BMJ 312(7032):670–674

97. Bowling A (1997) Rationing health care. Access to treatment should be equal, regardless of age. BMJ 314(7098):28

98. Wong DT, Gomez M, McGuire GP, Kavanagh B (1999) Utilization of intensive care unit days in a Canadian medical-surgical intensive care unit. Crit Care Med 27(7):1319–1324

99. Rapoport J, Lemeshow S, Le Gall J, Gehlbach S (1994) A method for assessing the clinical performance and cost-effectiveness of intensive care units: a multicenter inception cohort study. Crit Care Med 22(9):1385–1391

100. Eagle KA, Mulley AG, Skates SJ et al (1990) Length of stay in the intensive care unit. Effects of practice guidelines and feedback. Jama 264(8):992–997

101. Barnett R, Shustack A (1994) Cost containment: the Americas. Canada. New Horizons 2(3):332–335

102. Marcin JP, Slonim AD, Pollack MM, Ruttimann UE (2001) Long-stay patients in the pediatric intensive care unit. Crit Care Med 29(3):652–657

103. Slonim AD, Marcin JP, Pollack MM (2003) Long-stay patients: are there any long-term solutions? Crit Care Med 31(1):313–314

104. Rosenberg AL, Zimmerman JE, Alzola C et al (2000) Intensive care unit length of stay: recent changes and future challenges. Crit Care Med 28(10):3465–3473

105. Turnbull AD, Carlon G, Baron R et al (1979) The inverse relationship between cost and survival in the critically ill cancer patient. Crit Care Med 7(1):20–23

106. Detsky AS, Stricker SC, Mulley AG, Thibault GE (1981) Prognosis, survival, and the expenditure of hospital resources for patients in an intensive-care unit. N Engl J Med 305(12):667–672

107. Schroeder SA, Showstack JA, Roberts HE (1979) Frequency and clinical description of high-cost patients in 17 acute-care hospitals. N Engl J Med 300(23):1306–1309

108. Zook CJ, Moore FD (1980) High-cost users of medical care. N Engl J Med;302(18):996–1002

109. Welton JM, Meyer AA, Mandelkehr L et al (2002) Outcomes of and resource consumption by high-cost patients in the intensive care unit. Am J Crit Care 11(5):467–473

110. Madoff RD, Sharpe SM, Fath JJ et al (1985) Prolonged surgical intensive care. A useful allocation of medical resources. Arch Surg 120(6):698–702
111. Goins WA, Reynolds HN, Nyanjom D, Dunham CM (1991) Outcome following prolonged intensive care unit stay in multiple trauma patients. Crit Care Med 19(3):339–345
112. Cullen DJ, Ferrara LC, Briggs BA et al (1976) Survival, hospitalization charges and follow-up results in critically ill patients. N Engl J Med 294(18):982–987
113. Zaren B, Hedstrand U (1987) Quality of life among long-term survivors of intensive care. Crit Care Med 15(8):743–747
114. Ridley SA, Wallace PG (1990) Quality of life after intensive care. Anaesthesia 45(10):808–813
115. Niskanen M, Ruokonen E, Takala J et al (1999) Quality of life after prolonged intensive care. Crit Care Med 27(6):1132–1139
116. Eddy DM (1993) Clinical decision making: from theory to practice. Broadening the responsibilities of practitioners. The team approach. JAMA 269(14):1849–1855
117. Suter P, Armaganidis A, Beaufils F et al (1994) Predicting outcome in ICU patients. 2nd European Consensus Conference in Intensive Care Medicine. Intensive Care Med 20(5):390–397
118. Lipsett PA, Swoboda SM, Dickerson J et al (2000) Survival and functional outcome after prolonged intensive care unit stay. Annals of Surgery 231(2):262–268
119. Thoner J (1987) Outcome and costs of intensive care. A follow-up study on patients requiring prolonged mechanical ventilation. Acta Anaesthesiol Scand 31(8):693–698
120. Bone RC (1995) Economic analysis of the intensive care unit: a dilemma. Crit Care Med 23(5):805
121. Bone RC, McElwee NE, Eubanks DH, Gluck EH (1993) Analysis of indications for intensive care unit admission. Clinical efficacy assessment project: American College of Physicians. Chest 104(6):1806–1811
122. Rie M, Glessner T (1999) Best cost and best value budgeting for ICU respiratory readmissions. Crit Care Med 27:A48
123. Cooper GS, Sirio CA, Rotondi AJ et al (1999) Are readmissions to the intensive care unit a useful measure of hospital performance? Medical Care 37(4):399–408
124. Dobb GJ (1997) Intensive care in Australia and New Zealand. No nonsense 'down under'. Crit Care Clin 13(2):299–316
125. Angus DC, Sirio CA, Clermont G, Bion J (1997) International comparisons of critical care outcome and resource consumption. Crit Care Clin 13(2):389–407

GALLERY 2002 – 2005
After Affiliation of APICE to WFSICCM

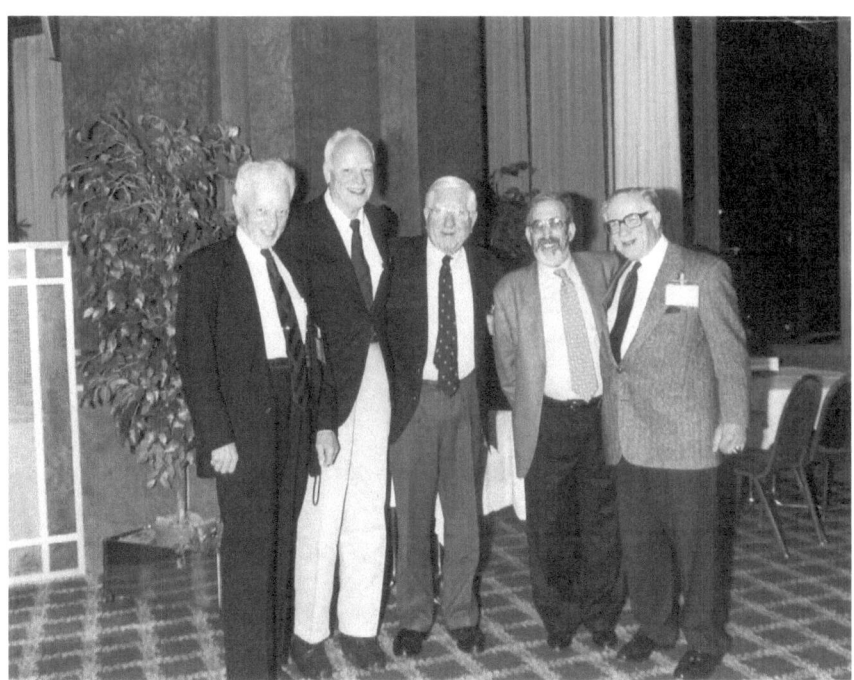

Left to right: P. Safar (USA), W.C. Shoemaker (USA), A.E. Baue (USA), A. Gullo (Italy), M.H. Weil (USA); Trieste, APICE 1998

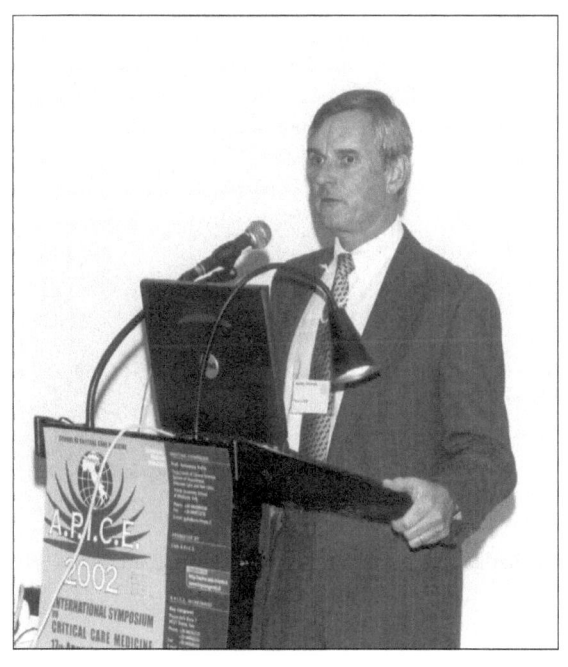

P.D. Lumb (USA); Trieste, APICE 2002

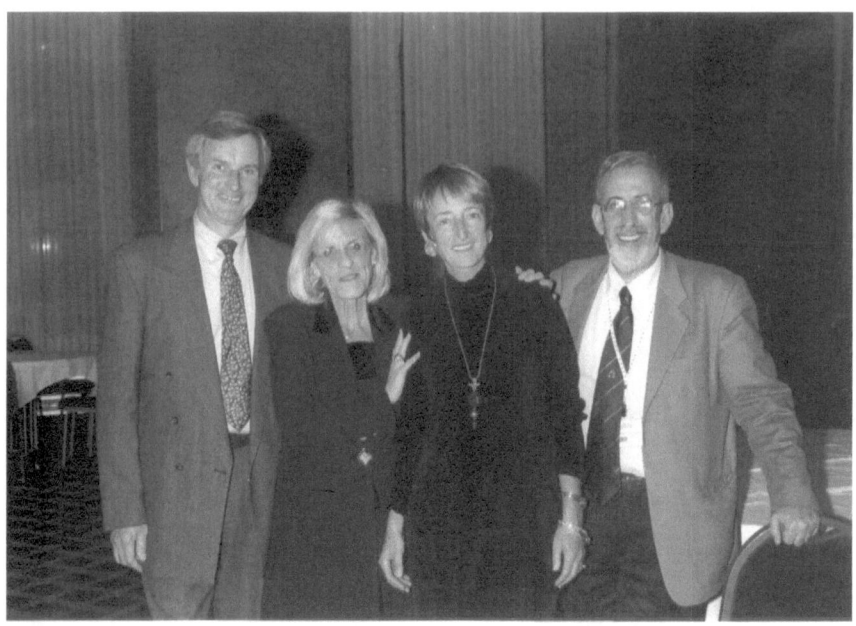

Left to right: P.D. Lumb (USA), D. Gullo (Italy), C. Lumb (USA), A. Gullo (Italy); Trieste, APICE 2002

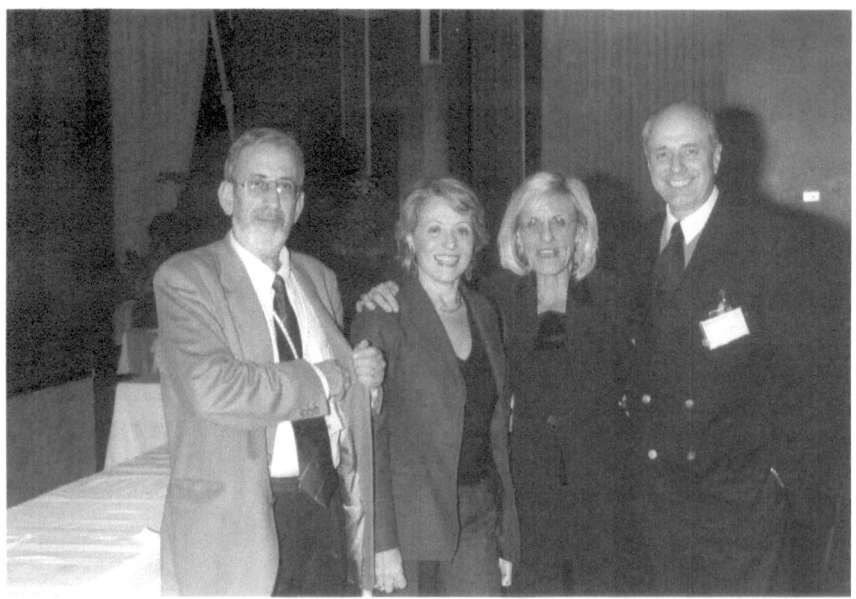

Left to right: A. Gullo (Italy), E. Muchada (France), D. Gullo (Italy), R. Muchada (France); Trieste, APICE 2002

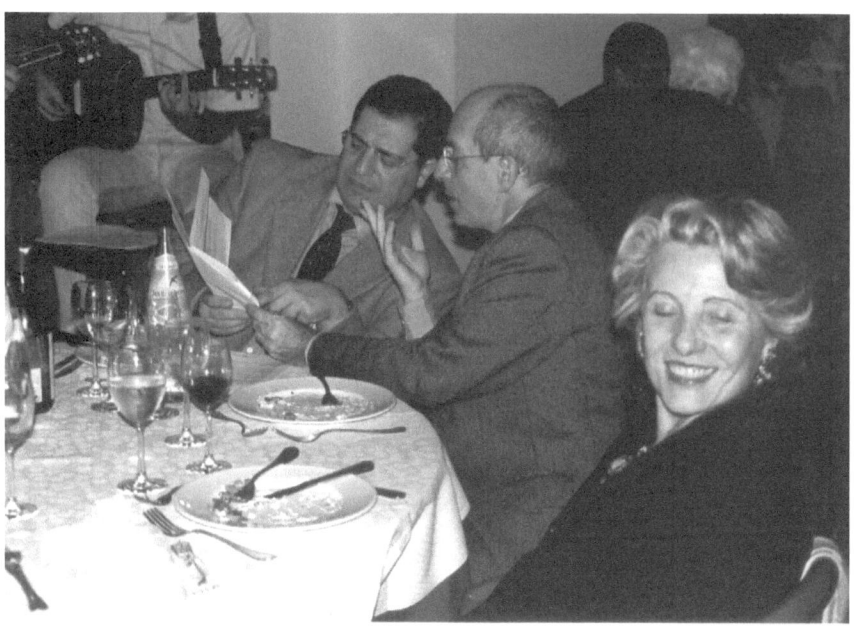

Left to right: G. Sganga (Italy), G. Berlot (Italy), E. Muchada (France); Trieste, APICE 2002

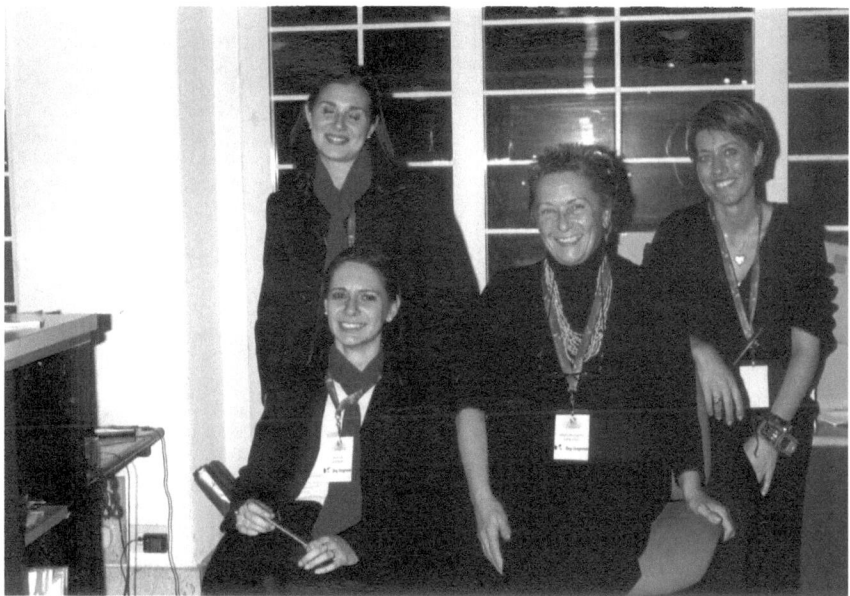

Left to right: O. Calamita (Italy), M. Gherbaz (Italy), M.N. Kravos (Italy), S. Tellini (Italy); Trieste, APICE Staff 2002

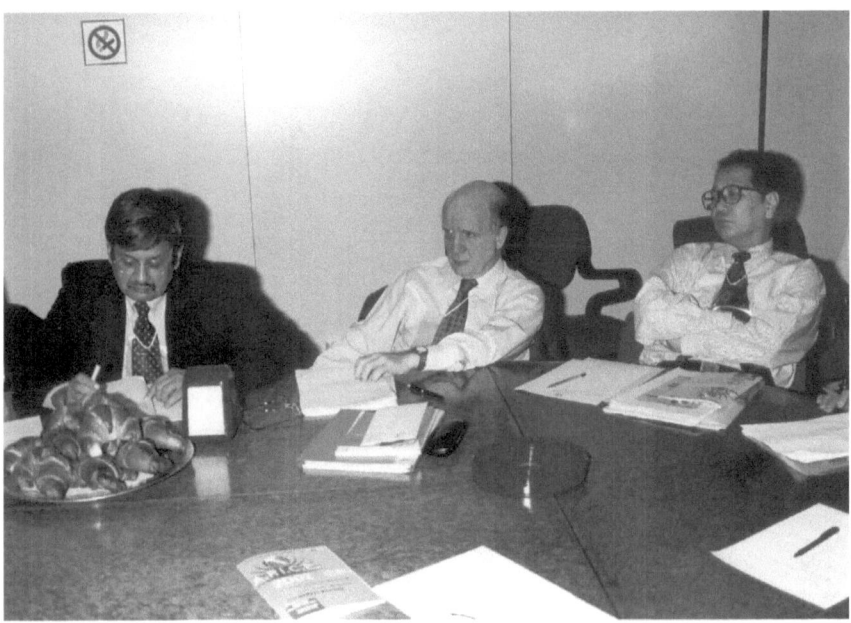

Left to right: S. Prayag (India), A. Gallesio (Argentina), J. Takezawa (Japan); Trieste, APICE 2002

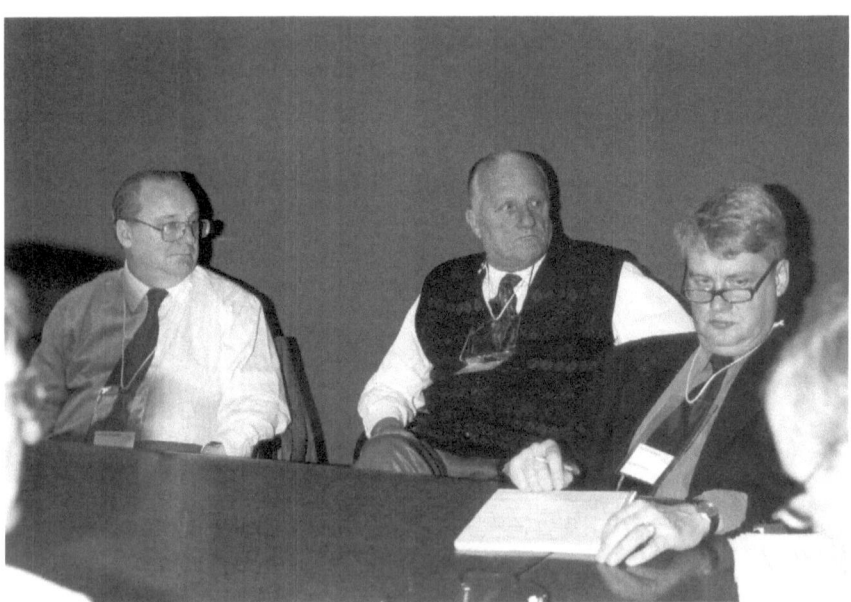

Left to right: F. Palizas (Argentina), R.G.G. Terzi (Brazil), L. Berggren (Sweden); Trieste, WFSICCM Council, APICE 2002

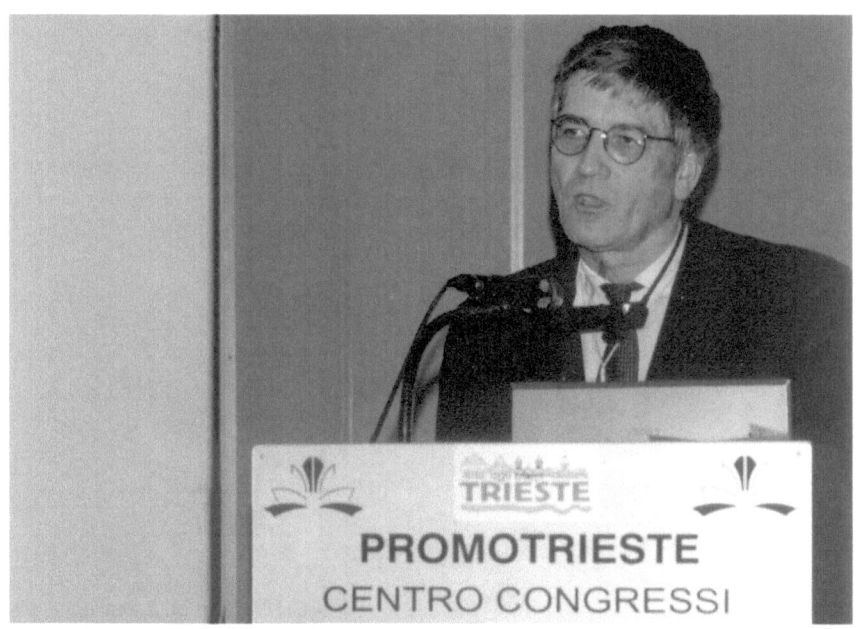

G. Park (UK); Trieste, APICE 2002

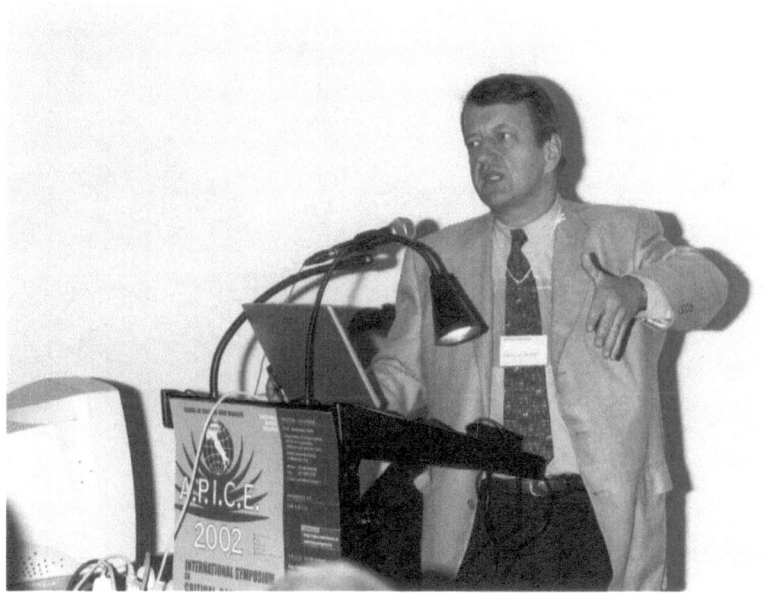

J.-L. Vincent (Belgium); Trieste, APICE 2002

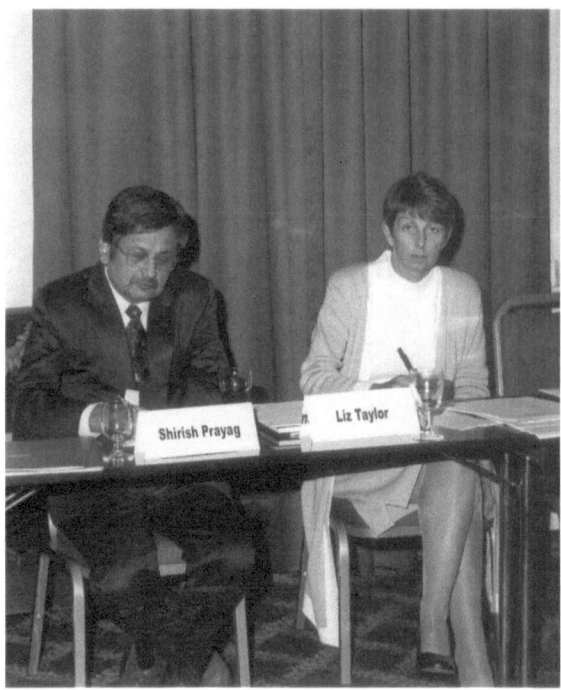

Left to right: S. Prayag (India), L. Taylor (UK); Trieste, WFSICCM Council, APICE 2002

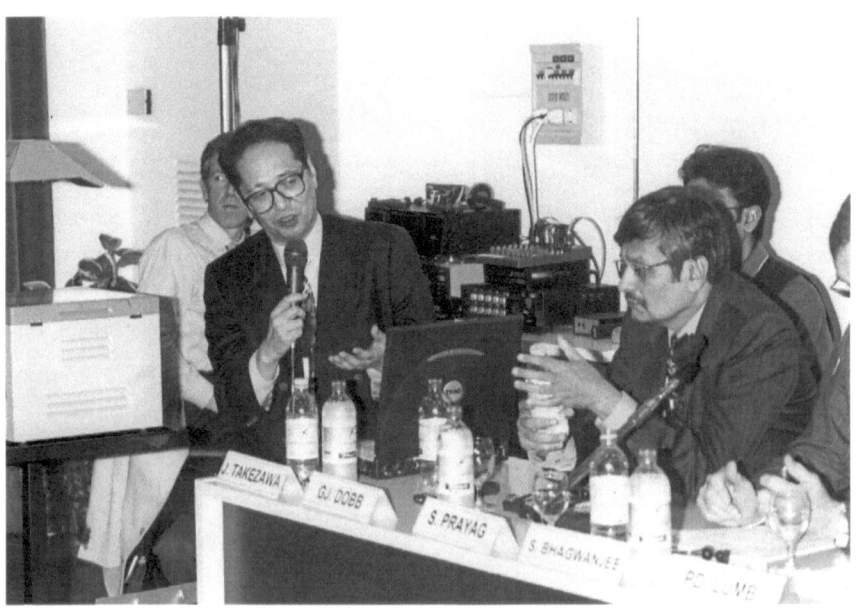

Left to right: J. Takezawa (Japan), S. Prayag (India); Trieste, APICE 2002

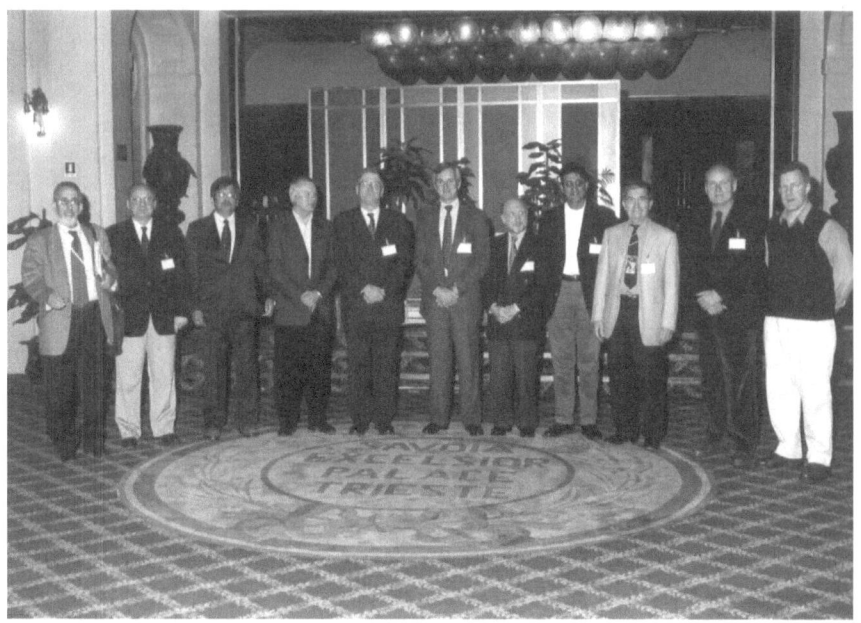

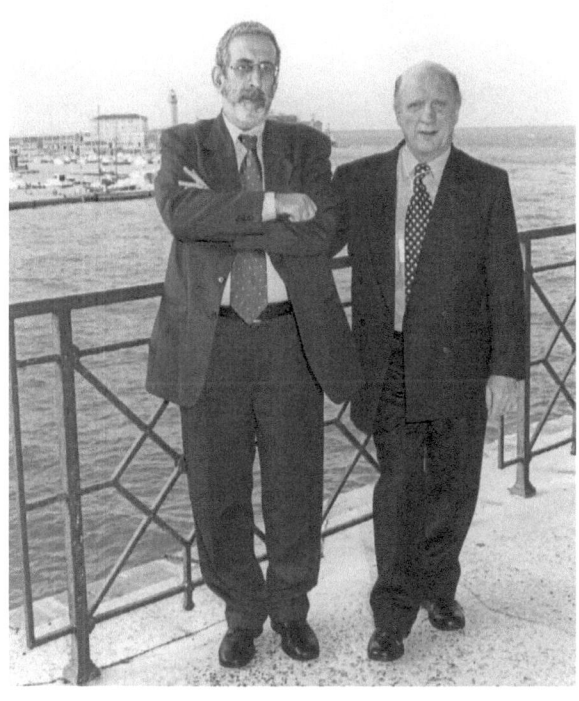

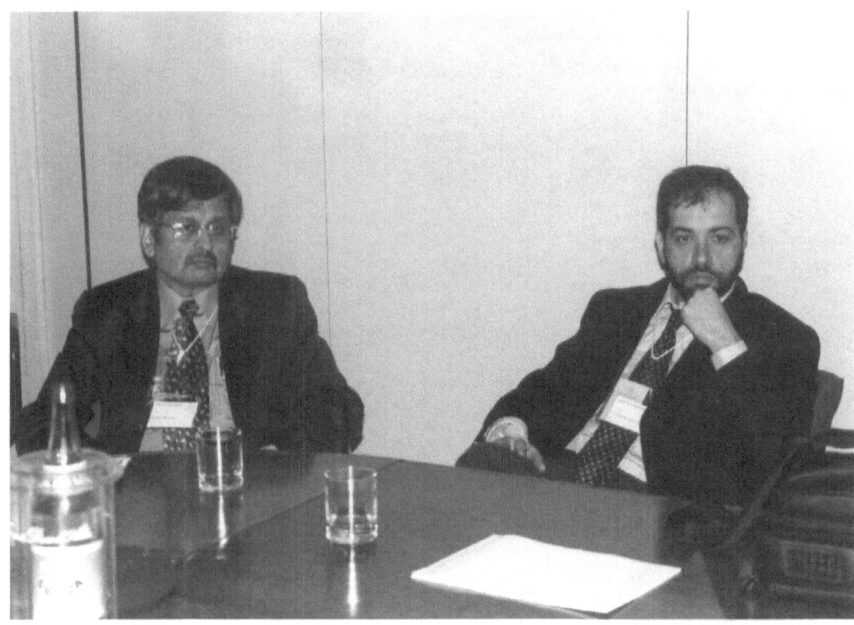

Left to right: S. Prayag (India), G. Dominguez-Cherit (Mexico); Trieste, APICE 2003

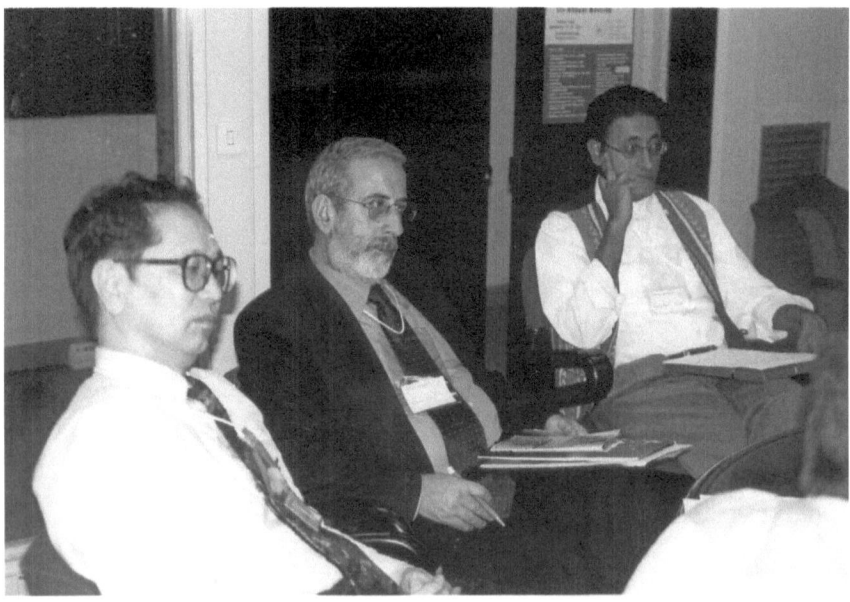

Left to right: J. Takezawa (Japan), A. Gullo (Italy), S. Bhagwanjee (South Africa); Trieste, WFSICCM Council, APICE 2003

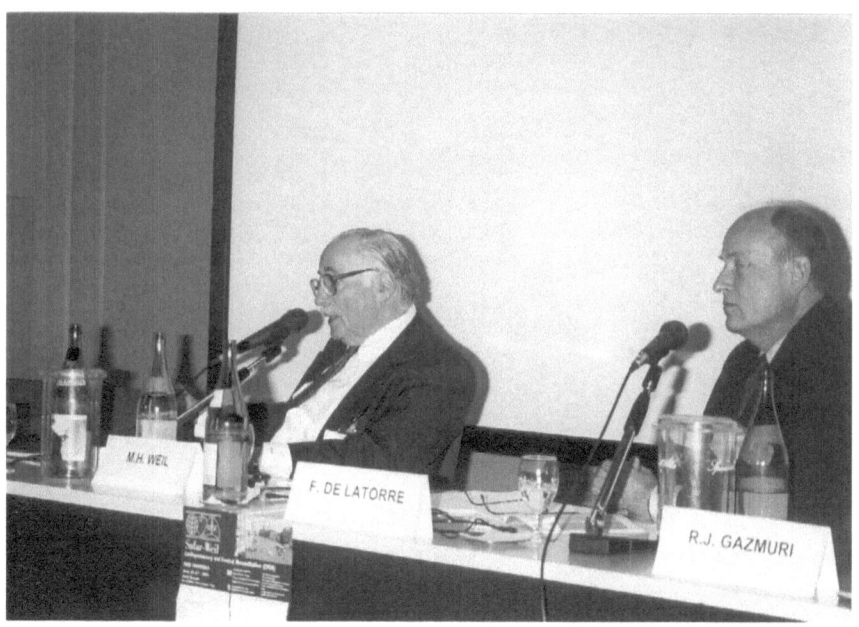

Left to right: M.H. Weil (USA), F. de Latorre (Spain); Trieste, APICE 2003

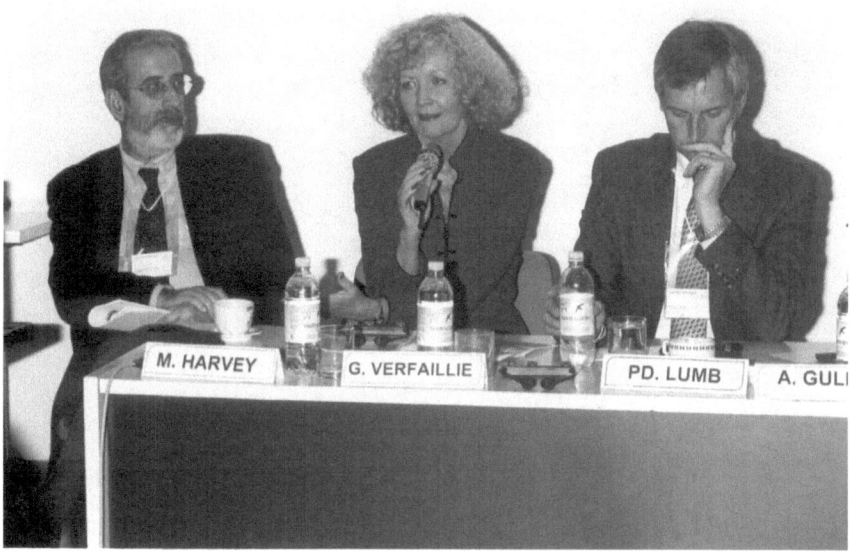

Left to right: A. Gullo (Italy), M. Harvey (USA), P.D. Lumb (USA); Trieste, APICE 2003

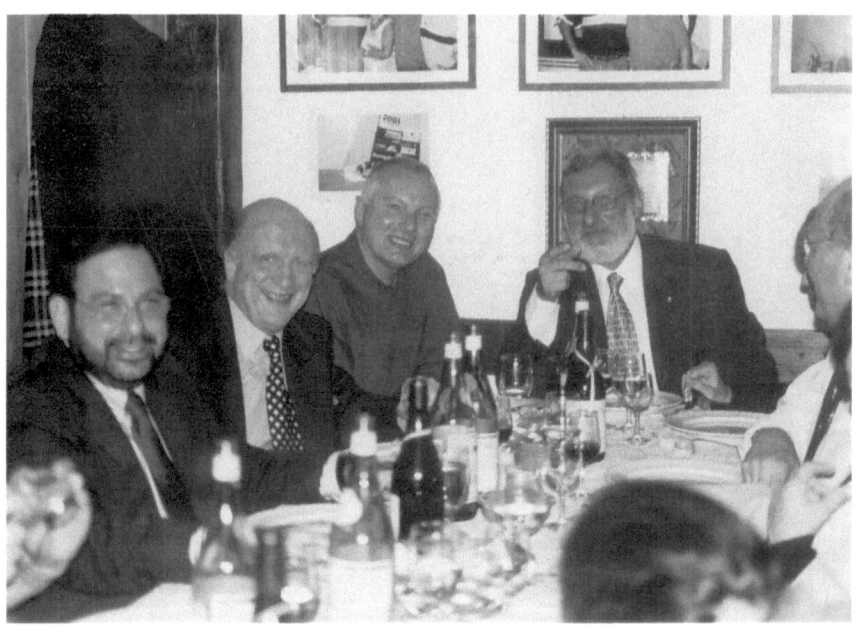

Left to right: J. Besso (Venezuela), A. Gallesio (Argentina), G.J. Dobb (Australia), G. Gurman (Israel); Trieste, APICE 2003

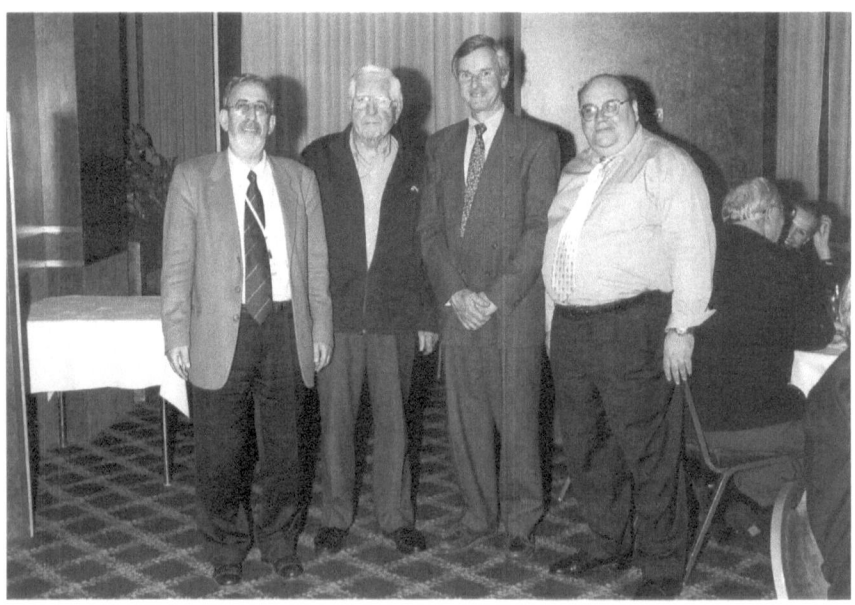

Left to right: A. Gullo (Italy), A.E. Baue (USA), P.D. Lumb (USA), E. Cohen (USA); Trieste, APICE 2003

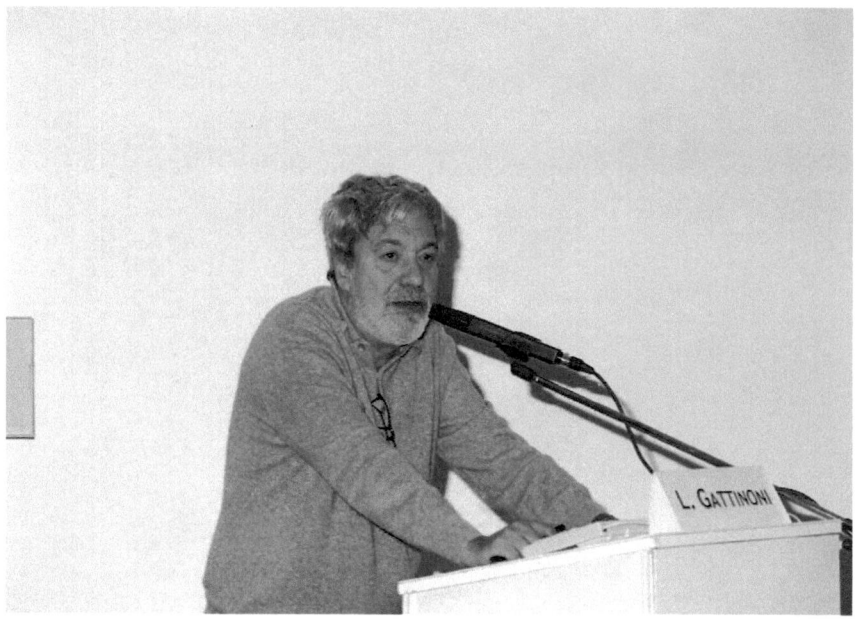

L. Gattinoni (Italy); Trieste, APICE 2004

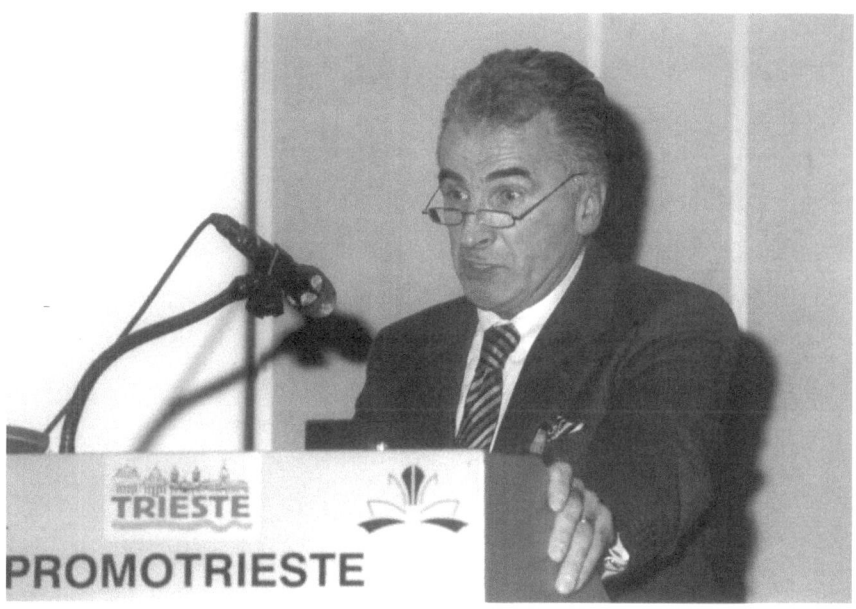

E. Nicolayenko (Russia); Trieste, APICE 2004

SUBJECT INDEX